THE SCIENCE-BACKED
AUTOIMMUNE
PROTOCOL
DIET FOR WOMEN

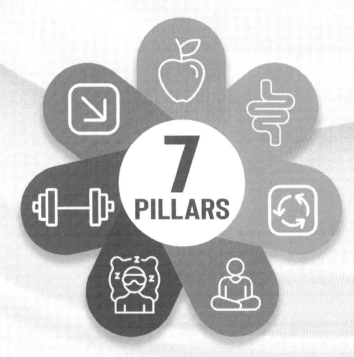

7 PILLARS

The 7 Essential Pillars to Restore Your
Immune System, Optimize Gut Health,
and Feel Your Best in 60 Days

ELIZA STONE

TABLE OF CONTENTS

A Personal Journey:
Understanding Autoimmune Diseases in Women

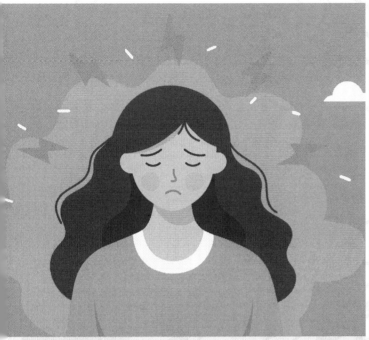

I remember the day I first experienced a surge of unexplainable fatigue and joint pain. Like so many women, I shrugged it off as stress or perhaps a side effect of balancing work, family, and daily responsibilities. But as time went on, the symptoms persisted, becoming more intense and widespread. My skin started flaring up unexpectedly, my digestion became erratic, and I began to feel a mental fog that made even simple decisions feel overwhelming. I felt as though my body had betrayed me, but it was more than that—it was a cry for help, signaling that something deeper was at play. It was the beginning of my journey with autoimmune disease.

Autoimmune diseases disproportionately affect women, with nearly 80% of autoimmune patients being female. This staggering statistic is not coincidental but is rooted in a complex interplay of genetic, hormonal, and environmental factors that uniquely impact women. Scientists and medical professionals are beginning to uncover the reasons behind this gender disparity, offering us not just insight but also a roadmap for managing these conditions.

The Gendered Nature of Autoimmunity

Autoimmune diseases, including rheumatoid arthritis, lupus, Hashimoto's thyroiditis, multiple sclerosis, and inflammatory bowel diseases, involve the immune system mistakenly attacking the body's own tissues. Researchers believe that the gender differences in autoimmune prevalence arise from both our biological and environmental landscapes. For women, hormonal fluctuations, particularly those related to estrogen, appear to play a significant role. Estrogen is known to have a stimulating effect on the immune system. While this can be protective against infections, it can also amplify the immune response, potentially leading to autoimmunity.

Moreover, the female immune system is generally more robust and responsive than that of males, which can paradoxically make women more susceptible to developing autoimmune conditions. During pregnancy, for example, a woman's immune system adjusts to tolerate the presence of a developing fetus, which is genetically distinct from her own body. This immunological flexibility is critical for reproduction but can sometimes result in dysregulation, especially if the immune system does not "reset" properly post-pregnancy.

In addition to these biological factors, the societal and psychological pressures placed on women can exacerbate the risk of autoimmunity. Women are often primary caregivers, managing both their households and careers, and this chronic stress can trigger or worsen autoimmune symptoms. Stress is known to affect the immune system by increasing the production of inflammatory cytokines, leading to a heightened state of immune reactivity. This is particularly relevant in autoimmune diseases, where the body is already primed for an overactive immune response.

Recognizing the Early Signs: When to Listen to Your Body

One of the most challenging aspects of autoimmune diseases is recognizing the symptoms early on. For many women, these symptoms manifest in subtle ways—lingering fatigue, muscle aches, bloating, skin rashes, or brain fog. It's easy to dismiss these as part of the "normal" stress of everyday life. However, the onset of autoimmune diseases is often insidious, with symptoms gradually building in intensity. By the time many women seek help, they have often experienced years of intermittent discomfort, testing their resilience and patience.

It's crucial to listen to our bodies and acknowledge these early warning signs. Autoimmune diseases are known for their periods of flare-ups and remissions, creating a false sense of recovery in between bouts. This cyclical nature can make it even harder to pinpoint a pattern, leading many women to feel as though they are at the mercy of their bodies.

My Personal Turning Point

For me, the turning point came when I realized that my symptoms were not just "in my head" or due to being overworked. After multiple doctor visits and a range of inconclusive tests, I was finally referred to a specialist who considered the possibility of an autoimmune condition. I underwent a battery of tests that eventually led to a diagnosis. While having a name for what was happening to my body provided some relief, it also brought with it a cascade of new questions and fears. How would this affect my life? Could I continue to be the mother, partner, and professional I aspired to be?

Embracing Knowledge as a Tool for Healing

Receiving an autoimmune diagnosis can be both empowering and terrifying. On one hand, it provides clarity and direction; on the other, it underscores the reality of living with a chronic condition. This is when I turned to research, driven by a need to understand my body and how I could regain control over my health. I discovered the Autoimmune Protocol (AIP) diet, a dietary regimen specifically designed to reduce inflammation, support gut health, and modulate the immune system.

In my quest for healing, I learned that the AIP diet's foundation lies in removing foods that may trigger the immune system and exacerbate symptoms. But beyond dietary changes, I also began to explore lifestyle factors—stress management, sleep, and physical activity—that could impact my autoimmune condition. It was through this multifaceted approach that I started to see improvements, slowly but surely. This journey wasn't just about food; it was about nurturing every aspect of my health, body, and mind.

Connecting with Other Women

One of the most eye-opening aspects of my journey was discovering the community of women who were also navigating the complexities of autoimmune diseases. Through online forums, support groups, and social media, I found countless stories of women with similar experiences—stories of struggle, resilience, and hope. We shared tips, recipes, setbacks, and victories. It was in these interactions that I realized I was not alone, and neither are you.

The journey with an autoimmune disease is deeply personal, and yet it is also collective. As women, we often carry the weight of our families, careers, and personal lives on our shoulders, all while managing our health in silence. But our stories matter. They are not just anecdotal experiences but crucial pieces of evidence that help build a more nuanced understanding of autoimmune diseases in women.

Your Journey Starts Here

This book is my way of reaching out to you, to provide not just information but also the encouragement and support I found so invaluable. It's about empowering you to take charge of your health through knowledge, science, and community. In the chapters that follow, we will dive into the science behind the AIP diet, uncovering how each element can restore balance to your immune system, optimize gut health, and, most importantly, help you feel like yourself again.

Whether you are at the beginning of your journey, seeking a diagnosis, or looking for new ways to manage your symptoms, this book is designed to guide you. I've walked this path, and while I don't have all the answers, I know that informed action is the key to reclaiming your life from autoimmunity.

This is your journey to healing—let's take the first step together.

Introduction

THE SCIENCE BEHIND HEALING: WHY THE AIP DIET WORKS

Autoimmune diseases can feel like an unwelcome invasion, where your own immune system has turned against you, mistaking your body's tissues as threats. What makes the Autoimmune Protocol (AIP) diet so powerful is that it addresses the root causes of this imbalance by restoring order to your immune system. This chapter will explore the scientific mechanisms behind the AIP diet and why it is especially effective for women who suffer from autoimmune conditions.

The Immune System's Role in Autoimmunity

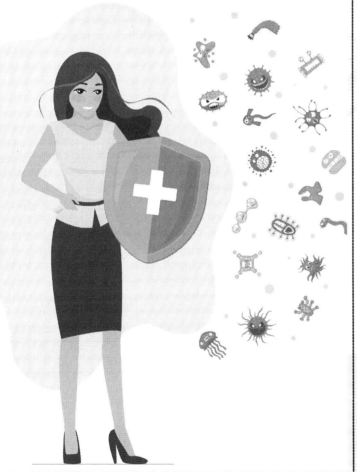

To understand how the AIP diet works, it's essential first to grasp what happens when the immune system goes awry. Normally, the immune system is designed to protect us by identifying and attacking foreign invaders, such as viruses and bacteria. It differentiates between what is "self" (our own tissues) and "non-self" (pathogens) through a sophisticated network of cells and signaling molecules.

However, in autoimmune diseases, this self-regulatory system breaks down. The immune system begins to attack its own cells, leading to chronic inflammation and tissue damage. This faulty immune response is often triggered or exacerbated by factors such as diet, stress, infections, and hormonal imbalances. For women, hormonal fluctuations related to menstrual cycles, pregnancy, and menopause can further alter immune function, increasing their susceptibility to autoimmune conditions.

The AIP diet works by addressing three key areas that directly impact the immune system: gut health, inflammation, and food sensitivities. Let's delve into the science of how each of these factors plays a role in autoimmunity and how the AIP diet helps correct them.

1. Healing the Gut: The Foundation of Immunity

The health of your gut, or gastrointestinal (GI) tract, is crucial for a well-functioning immune system. In fact, around 70% of the immune system resides in the gut-associated lymphoid tissue (GALT). A healthy gut acts as a barrier, preventing harmful substances, pathogens, and toxins from entering the bloodstream. This barrier is maintained by tightly connected cells lining the intestinal wall, known as tight junctions.

However, in individuals with autoimmune diseases, these tight junctions often become compromised, leading to a condition commonly referred to as "leaky gut." Scientifically known as increased intestinal permeability, leaky gut allows undigested food particles, toxins, and microbes to pass through the gut lining into the bloodstream. Once these foreign particles enter the bloodstream, they can trigger an immune response, leading to chronic inflammation and potentially setting off a cascade of autoimmune reactions.

The AIP diet specifically targets gut healing by eliminating foods that are known to irritate the gut lining and promote permeability. Gluten, found in grains like wheat, rye, and barley, is a known culprit for increasing gut permeability, particularly in genetically predisposed individuals. Other foods, such as nightshades (tomatoes, peppers, eggplants), legumes, and certain food additives, can also irritate the gut and exacerbate inflammation. By removing these foods, the AIP diet helps the gut lining to repair itself, restoring its ability to function as a proper barrier.

Moreover, the AIP diet emphasizes the consumption of nutrient-dense foods that are rich in vitamins, minerals, and antioxidants, such as leafy greens, bone broth, and organ meats. These foods supply the body with the building blocks needed to regenerate the gut lining, reduce inflammation, and promote the growth of beneficial gut bacteria. A healthy microbiome is integral to gut health, as it plays a critical role in regulating immune responses and maintaining intestinal barrier integrity. Recent studies have shown that dietary changes, like those promoted by the AIP diet, can positively alter the gut microbiome, leading to improved immune regulation and reduced autoimmune symptoms.

2. Reducing Chronic Inflammation: The Root of Autoimmune Flare-ups

Chronic inflammation is a hallmark of autoimmune diseases. When the immune system mistakenly attacks the body's tissues, it releases inflammatory molecules called cytokines. While short-term inflammation is a protective mechanism, chronic inflammation can result in tissue damage, pain, and a host of other symptoms associated with autoimmunity.

The foods eliminated in the AIP diet, such as grains, dairy, refined sugars, and processed foods, are known to promote inflammation in various ways. For example, refined sugars and processed foods can spike blood sugar levels, leading to insulin resistance and increased production of inflammatory cytokines. Grains, especially those containing gluten, can activate inflammatory pathways in the body, further aggravating autoimmune conditions.

The AIP diet works to calm this inflammation by focusing on anti-inflammatory, nutrient-rich foods. For example, foods like oily fish (salmon, mackerel) and grass-fed meats are high in omega-3 fatty acids, which have been shown to reduce inflammation and modulate immune responses. Additionally, the AIP diet includes an abundance of vegetables, rich in phytonutrients and antioxidants that combat oxidative stress, a key player in chronic inflammation.

In women, hormonal fluctuations can exacerbate inflammation, particularly during menstruation, pregnancy, and menopause. The AIP diet's emphasis on balancing blood sugar levels, reducing gut inflammation, and providing ample nutrients supports hormonal balance. By creating a less inflammatory internal environment, the body can better regulate its immune response and reduce the intensity of autoimmune flare-ups.

3. Identifying and Eliminating Food Sensitivities

Food sensitivities and intolerances play a significant role in autoimmunity, acting as ongoing triggers for the immune system. Unlike food allergies, which provoke an immediate immune response, food sensitivities cause delayed reactions, making them harder to identify. Symptoms can manifest as digestive issues, joint pain, skin rashes, or fatigue—symptoms that are often mistaken for other conditions or overlooked entirely.

The elimination phase of the AIP diet is designed to identify these hidden food sensitivities by removing common trigger foods and gradually reintroducing them one at a time. During the elimination phase, foods that are known to cause immune system activation—such as dairy, eggs, nuts, seeds, and nightshades—are excluded. This approach allows the body to reset and reduces the overall immune burden.

After a period of healing, foods are reintroduced methodically to observe how the body reacts. This process not only helps identify individual food triggers but also empowers women to make informed dietary choices based on their unique biological responses. Research suggests that such personalized dietary interventions can be highly effective in reducing autoimmune symptoms and achieving long-term remission.

Why the AIP Diet Is Particularly Effective for Women

For women, the AIP diet provides a targeted strategy to address the unique physiological and hormonal factors that contribute to autoimmune diseases. Women's immune systems are inherently more responsive, which, while advantageous in fighting infections, can also make them more prone to autoimmune responses. By reducing dietary triggers, calming inflammation, and supporting gut health, the AIP diet helps modulate this heightened immune activity.

Additionally, the AIP diet encourages the consumption of foods that support hormonal health, such as healthy fats, nutrient-rich vegetables, and anti-inflammatory proteins. These dietary choices can help stabilize hormones, reduce stress on the body, and support energy levels, addressing many of the specific concerns women have when managing autoimmune conditions.

The Evidence Speaks

Emerging research continues to support the effectiveness of the AIP diet in managing autoimmune diseases. Clinical studies have shown that patients with autoimmune conditions such as inflammatory bowel disease (IBD) and Hashimoto's thyroiditis experienced significant symptom reduction, improved quality of life, and reduced inflammatory markers after following the AIP diet. While more research is needed to fully understand the mechanisms at play, these findings underscore the potential of the AIP diet as a science-backed approach to healing.

By taking a comprehensive approach that addresses gut health, reduces inflammation, and identifies food sensitivities, the AIP diet provides women with a powerful tool to reclaim their health. It's not just about what you eat; it's about nourishing your body in a way that allows your immune system to find its balance once again. The science behind the AIP diet offers hope and a clear pathway toward feeling your best in 60 days and beyond.

YOUR 60-DAY TRANSFORMATION: HOW TO USE THIS BOOK FOR OPTIMAL RESULTS

Embarking on a journey to regain your health and well-being can feel overwhelming, especially when facing the complexities of autoimmune diseases. The next 60 days will be pivotal in transforming not just your diet, but also your lifestyle, mindset, and overall approach to managing your condition. This chapter is designed to provide a clear, science-backed roadmap to help you use this book effectively, maximize the benefits of the Autoimmune Protocol (AIP) diet, and support your body's natural healing processes. With each day, you will build momentum, creating sustainable habits that will support your health for the long term.

The 60-Day Framework: Why 60 Days?

Why 60 days, you may ask? The immune system and gut health require time to reset and restore balance. Research shows that significant dietary changes often need a consistent period to fully manifest their benefits, especially in the context of chronic conditions like autoimmune diseases. A 60-day window is long enough to allow your body to begin the process of gut repair, immune modulation, and reduction of chronic inflammation.

In this timeframe, you will go through several critical phases: an initial detoxification as you eliminate inflammatory foods, a stabilization phase as your body adjusts to nutrient-dense eating, and an initial reintroduction period where you can begin to identify which foods support your health and which do not. By following this structured approach, you'll be setting yourself up for both short-term relief and long-term management of your symptoms.

Getting Started: Preparing for Success

Before diving into the detailed plan, it's crucial to prepare both mentally and practically. Studies indicate that mindset and preparation play a significant role in the success of any dietary intervention. Here's how to set the stage for a successful 60-day transformation:

1. Set Clear Goals:

Define your personal goals for the next 60 days. Whether it's reducing joint pain, improving energy levels, or gaining mental clarity, having a clear set of intentions will help you stay focused. Write these goals down, as research suggests that documenting intentions can significantly increase the likelihood of achieving them.

2. Track Your Baseline:

It's essential to establish a baseline before starting your journey. Note your current symptoms, energy levels, digestive health, and mental state. You can use the health journal template in the appendix to record details. Tracking these aspects will provide you with tangible evidence of your progress throughout the 60 days, motivating you to continue and adjust as necessary.

3. Stock Your Kitchen:

The AIP diet requires specific ingredients to create nourishing, inflammation-reducing meals. Research shows that a well-stocked kitchen is linked to better adherence to dietary changes. Refer to the grocery list in Chapter 14 to ensure you have everything you need. Preparing your kitchen in advance will make the transition into AIP-friendly cooking smoother and less stressful.

4. Create a Support System:

Inform your family and close friends about your 60-day plan. Social support has been shown to significantly improve success rates in lifestyle changes, particularly those involving diet and health. Consider joining an online AIP support group or finding a health coach or nutritionist who specializes in autoimmune protocols for additional guidance and encouragement.

The 60-Day Journey: A Week-by-Week Guide

The next 60 days are divided into manageable weekly segments, each with a focus to guide you through the various stages of the AIP diet. This book includes weekly objectives, meal plans, lifestyle strategies, and reflection points to help you stay on track.

Weeks 1-2: The Initial Transition (Days 1-14)

The first two weeks are crucial for eliminating the primary food triggers and transitioning to nutrient-dense, anti-inflammatory meals. This period involves detoxifying your body from foods that may have been contributing to your symptoms, such as gluten, dairy, processed sugars, and nightshades. Scientifically, it can take 1-2 weeks for inflammatory cytokines triggered by these foods to begin decreasing in the body.

- Focus: Eliminating inflammatory foods and introducing healing, nutrient-dense alternatives.
- Key Actions:
  - Follow the detailed elimination guide in Chapter 5.
  - Use the provided meal plans in Chapter 12 to ease into AIP-compliant cooking.
- Self-Care: These weeks may come with some withdrawal symptoms like fatigue or cravings. Implement the stress-reduction techniques outlined in Chapter 9 to help your body adjust.

Weeks 3-4: Finding Your Rhythm (Days 15-28)

By now, your body will have started to adapt to the new dietary changes. The focus during this phase is to solidify your meal-prepping habits, diversify your nutrient intake, and continue supporting gut health.

- Focus: Building consistency and enhancing gut healing.
- Key Actions:
  - Experiment with new AIP recipes to keep your meals exciting and diverse.
  - Introduce gut-healing foods such as bone broth, fermented vegetables, and omega-3-rich fish, as outlined in Chapter 7.
- Reflection: Use your health journal to document changes in symptoms. Noticing even small improvements, such as better sleep or reduced bloating, will reinforce the positive impact of your dietary choices.

Weeks 5-6: Enhancing Lifestyle (Days 29-42)

At this point, you'll start to notice more tangible benefits, such as improved digestion, more consistent energy levels, and possibly a reduction in flare-ups. Now, it's time to integrate additional lifestyle elements that further support immune balance, including stress management, sleep optimization, and gentle physical activity.

- Focus: Incorporating lifestyle modifications to optimize healing.
- Key Actions:
  - Follow the sleep improvement strategies in Chapter 10 to enhance recovery and immune function.
  - Begin incorporating gentle, mind-body exercises, such as yoga or walking, as discussed in Chapter 11.
- Adjustment: If certain symptoms persist, use the troubleshooting section of Chapter 12 to identify potential issues and adapt your diet or lifestyle changes accordingly.

Weeks 7-8: The Reintroduction Phase (Days 43-60)

By now, you should have established a strong foundation of AIP-compliant eating and lifestyle habits. The final weeks focus on the careful reintroduction of foods to identify potential sensitivities. It is during this phase that you start to discover which foods you can reintroduce into your diet without triggering symptoms.

- Focus: Identifying food sensitivities and personalizing your diet.
- Key Actions:
  - Follow the reintroduction protocol in Chapter 8, starting with the foods you miss the most or those that are nutrient-dense.
  - Reintroduce one food at a time, allowing 5-7 days between each new introduction to monitor for any delayed reactions.
- Reflection: Record your body's responses to each reintroduced food in your journal. This information will be critical in customizing a long-term dietary plan that supports your unique needs.

Building Momentum: Tips for Sustained Success

As you progress through the 60 days, remember that this journey is not about perfection but about consistent effort and self-compassion. Here are a few science-backed strategies to help maintain your momentum:

- Celebrate Small Wins: Positive reinforcement is shown to boost motivation. Acknowledge every small step you take toward improved health, whether it's a day without pain, a new recipe tried, or a successful reintroduction.
- Adapt as Needed: Each woman's body is unique, and so will be your response to the AIP diet. Use the tracking tools provided in this book to fine-tune your approach based on your observations and results.

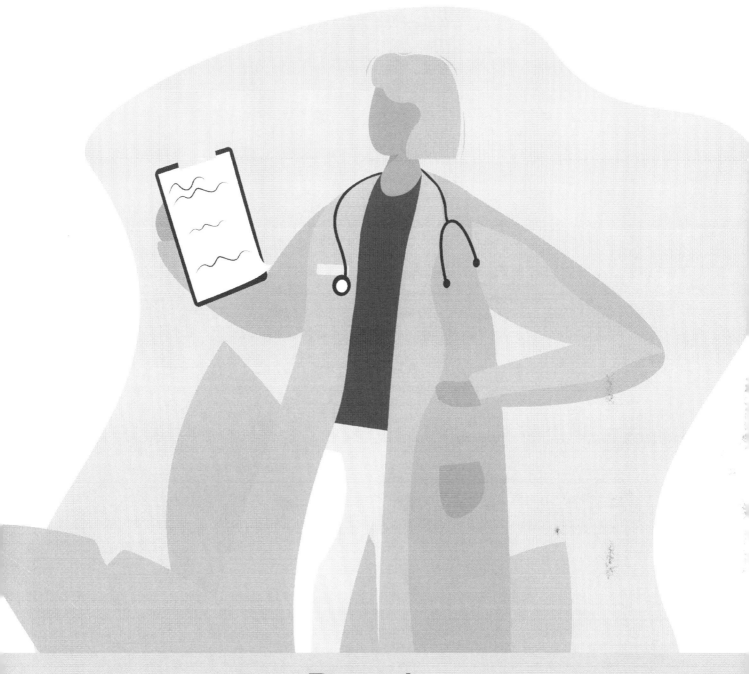

Part I:
Understanding Autoimmune Diseases and the AIP Diet

Chapter 1:
The Rise of Autoimmune Diseases in Women

In recent decades, autoimmune diseases have surged, disproportionately affecting women at a staggering rate. Currently, women account for nearly 80% of autoimmune cases, a trend that has puzzled researchers and healthcare professionals. Factors such as hormonal fluctuations, genetic predispositions, environmental triggers, and lifestyle changes have all been identified as potential contributors to this growing epidemic. Modern lifestyles, characterized by chronic stress, dietary changes, and increased exposure to toxins, have put the female immune system under immense pressure. As researchers continue to explore this phenomenon, it has become clear that autoimmune diseases in women are a complex interplay of biological, environmental, and societal factors. Understanding this rise is crucial for developing effective, science-backed strategies to manage and prevent these conditions. This chapter dives into the reasons behind the increase in autoimmune diseases among women, setting the stage for an informed approach to healing.

THE PREVALENCE OF AUTOIMMUNITY AMONG WOMEN

Autoimmune diseases have become a major health concern worldwide, with women bearing the brunt of this epidemic. Studies show that nearly 80% of autoimmune conditions, including lupus, rheumatoid arthritis, multiple sclerosis, and Hashimoto's thyroiditis, are diagnosed in women. While autoimmunity can develop at any age, women are most vulnerable during their reproductive years, suggesting a potential link between hormonal changes and immune function.

Scientists attribute this gender disparity to several biological and genetic factors. Women possess a more robust and responsive immune system compared to men, which is partly due to the influence of estrogen on immune cells. While this heightened immunity can offer protection against infections, it may also increase the risk of the immune system mistakenly attacking the body's own tissues. Additionally, specific genetic markers, such as variations in the X chromosome—which women have two copies of—are linked to a higher susceptibility to autoimmune diseases.

Environmental and lifestyle factors also play a crucial role. Women are more frequently exposed to certain triggers like chronic stress, chemical pollutants in personal care products, and dietary shifts, all of which can provoke immune dysregulation. Understanding these multifaceted reasons for the high prevalence of autoimmunity in women is essential for developing targeted strategies to mitigate the risk and manage symptoms effectively.

COMMON AUTOIMMUNE CONDITIONS AFFECTING WOMEN

Women are disproportionately affected by a variety of autoimmune diseases, many of which can lead to chronic pain, fatigue, and significantly impaired quality of life. Among the most prevalent are lupus, rheumatoid arthritis, Hashimoto's thyroiditis, multiple sclerosis (MS), and Sjögren's syndrome. These conditions are not only more common in women but often present with unique symptoms and patterns influenced by hormonal fluctuations, genetic factors, and immune system differences.

Lupus, or systemic lupus erythematosus (SLE), is one of the most well-known autoimmune diseases affecting women, with around 90% of patients being female. Lupus occurs when the immune system mistakenly attacks healthy tissues, leading to widespread inflammation in organs such as the skin, joints, kidneys, and heart. Estrogen has been found to modulate immune activity, potentially explaining why lupus flare-ups often coincide with menstrual cycles and pregnancy.

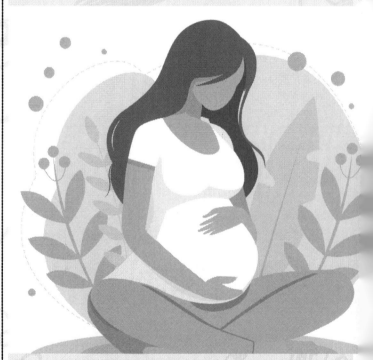

Rheumatoid arthritis (RA) primarily targets the synovial lining of joints, resulting in pain, swelling, and, over time, joint deformity. Women are three times more likely than men to develop RA, usually during their childbearing years. Research suggests that hormonal factors, such as elevated levels of prolactin, may contribute to the higher incidence in women. Environmental factors like smoking and diet can also play a role in the onset and severity of RA symptoms.

Hashimoto's thyroiditis is an autoimmune condition where the immune system attacks the thyroid gland, leading to hypothyroidism. This disease predominantly affects women, especially during periods of hormonal change, such as pregnancy, postpartum, and menopause. Hashimoto's is characterized by fatigue, weight gain, and sensitivity to cold, among other symptoms, all of which stem from reduced thyroid hormone production. Women with Hashimoto's often experience significant challenges in managing metabolism, mood, and energy levels.

Multiple sclerosis (MS) is another autoimmune disorder with a higher prevalence in women. MS targets the central nervous system, where the immune system damages the protective sheath (myelin) covering nerve fibers. The disease disrupts communication between the brain and the rest of the body, leading to symptoms ranging from muscle weakness to cognitive impairment. Recent studies suggest that the female hormone estradiol may influence the course of MS, with fluctuations possibly affecting the frequency and severity of relapses.

Sjögren's syndrome primarily impacts the moisture-producing glands, causing symptoms such as dry eyes and mouth. Like other autoimmune diseases, Sjögren's is significantly more common in women, with an estimated 9 out of 10 patients being female. The condition can occur on its own or in conjunction with other autoimmune disorders, such as rheumatoid arthritis or lupus, further complicating diagnosis and treatment.

These conditions illustrate the complex nature of autoimmunity in women. By understanding the specific characteristics and risk factors associated with these common autoimmune diseases, women can take informed steps towards managing their health, guided by strategies like the Autoimmune Protocol (AIP) diet to reduce inflammation and support immune regulation.

Chapter 2:
Decoding the Immune System

To effectively manage autoimmune diseases, it's crucial to understand how the immune system functions and, more importantly, what happens when it malfunctions. The immune system is a complex network of cells, tissues, and organs designed to protect the body from harmful invaders like bacteria, viruses, and toxins. In healthy individuals, this defense system can distinguish between "self" (the body's own cells) and "non-self" (foreign substances), launching a targeted attack only when necessary. However, in autoimmune conditions, this recognition process breaks down, causing the immune system to mistakenly target healthy tissues. For women, this misdirected attack can be influenced by unique factors, including hormonal changes, genetics, and environmental exposures. This chapter will explore the science of immune regulation, focusing on how the body's natural defenses can go awry in autoimmune diseases. By decoding these intricate processes, we can better grasp how dietary and lifestyle changes, like the AIP diet, can aid in restoring balance.

HOW A HEALTHY IMMUNE SYSTEM FUNCTIONS

The immune system is the body's frontline defense against pathogens, equipped with a sophisticated array of mechanisms to detect, respond to, and eliminate foreign invaders. It comprises two main components: the innate and adaptive immune systems. Together, they form a dynamic and highly coordinated response to keep the body protected.

The innate immune system serves as the body's first line of defense, acting rapidly upon encountering a potential threat. It includes physical barriers such as the skin and mucous membranes, as well as immune cells like macrophages, neutrophils, and natural killer cells. These cells identify pathogens through broad, non-specific markers, launching an immediate attack to prevent infection from spreading. The innate response also includes the release of cytokines, signaling proteins that help recruit other immune cells to the site of infection, intensifying the body's defense.

If the innate immune response is insufficient, the adaptive immune system steps in. Unlike the innate system, the adaptive immune system is highly specific. It involves T-cells and B-cells, which can recognize and remember specific antigens—unique molecular structures found on pathogens. Upon first exposure, the body creates a tailored immune response, producing antibodies through B-cells that can neutralize the invader. T-cells, on the other hand, can directly kill infected cells or help modulate the overall immune response. This adaptive memory is what allows the body to mount a faster, more effective defense upon subsequent encounters with the same pathogen.

Regulation is a key feature of a healthy immune system. Cells called regulatory T-cells (Tregs) play an essential role in maintaining balance, ensuring that the immune system does not overreact or mistakenly target the body's own tissues. Additionally, the gut is a central regulator of immune function; it houses nearly 70% of the body's immune cells and provides a crucial interface between the internal and external environments.

In women, hormonal fluctuations, particularly of estrogen and progesterone, can modulate immune activity. Estrogen generally enhances the immune response, increasing the production of antibodies and cytokines. While this can make women more effective at fighting off infections, it can also predispose them to a more active and, at times, dysregulated immune response. A healthy immune system is thus one that is vigilant but not overly aggressive—able to distinguish between harmful invaders and the body's own cells, maintaining equilibrium that is vital for overall well-being. Understanding this balance is crucial for managing autoimmune conditions, where the system mistakenly attacks its own tissues.

WHAT GOES WRONG: THE ONSET OF AUTOIMMUNITY

In autoimmune diseases, the body's carefully regulated immune system begins to malfunction, turning its defenses against its own tissues. This self-attack occurs when the immune system loses the ability to differentiate between "self" and "non-self," a process known as immune tolerance. Several factors contribute to this breakdown, resulting in the onset of autoimmunity, especially in women.

One of the central issues is molecular mimicry, a phenomenon where the immune system mistakes the body's cells for foreign invaders. This often happens after an infection; certain pathogens carry proteins that closely resemble those found in human tissues. When the immune system creates antibodies to combat the infection, these antibodies can inadvertently target the body's own cells, leading to autoimmune reactions.

Genetic predisposition plays a significant role as well. Women are more likely to carry specific genes associated with autoimmunity, such as variations in the HLA (human leukocyte antigen) complex. This complex is responsible for presenting antigens to immune cells, and alterations in its function can trigger an inappropriate immune response. The presence of two X chromosomes in women further contributes to genetic vulnerability, as the X chromosome contains many immune-related genes.

Hormonal fluctuations add another layer of complexity. Hormones like estrogen and progesterone directly influence immune cell activity. While estrogen generally enhances the immune response, it can also heighten the risk of immune dysregulation. This is evident in the higher rates of autoimmune disease onset during periods of hormonal change in women, such as puberty, pregnancy, postpartum, and menopause. These fluctuations can amplify the immune response, increasing the likelihood of mistargeting the body's tissues.

Lastly, environmental factors such as diet, stress, toxins, and infections can act as triggers. Poor gut health, characterized by increased intestinal permeability (often referred to as "leaky gut"), allows undigested food particles and toxins to enter the bloodstream, prompting an immune response. Over time, these repeated assaults can tip the immune system into a state of chronic inflammation, where it becomes hyper-responsive and prone to autoimmunity.

The onset of autoimmunity is thus a multifactorial process involving genetic, hormonal, and environmental components. This complex interplay disrupts the immune system's tolerance, resulting in a misguided attack on the body's own tissues. Understanding these mechanisms is crucial for implementing strategies like the Autoimmune Protocol (AIP) diet, which aims to reduce inflammation and support immune balance.

INFLAMMATION: FRIEND AND FOE

Inflammation is a critical function of the immune system, acting as a first responder when the body encounters injury, infection, or harmful stimuli. When functioning correctly, inflammation serves as a protective mechanism that helps to isolate and eliminate invaders while initiating the healing process. However, when inflammation becomes chronic, it turns from a friend into a foe, contributing to the development and progression of autoimmune diseases.

Acute inflammation is the body's way of responding to threats. When you cut your finger, for example, immune cells rush to the site, releasing signaling molecules called cytokines that dilate blood vessels, increase blood flow, and draw white blood cells to the area. This process results in redness, swelling, and warmth—hallmarks of acute inflammation—and is a sign that your body is actively fighting off potential infection and beginning the repair process. In this scenario, inflammation is both necessary and beneficial, promoting tissue healing and restoring balance.

However, problems arise when the inflammatory response does not shut down as it should. This chronic inflammation occurs when the immune system continues to release pro-inflammatory cytokines even in the absence of an actual threat. In autoimmune diseases, the immune system mistakenly identifies the body's own cells as harmful, perpetuating a cycle of ongoing inflammation. Over time, this chronic inflammation can lead to tissue damage and disrupt normal cellular functions, worsening symptoms.

For women, hormonal fluctuations can significantly influence the body's inflammatory response. Estrogen, which modulates immune activity, can increase the production of certain cytokines during various stages of the menstrual cycle. While this heightened immune activity can be advantageous in combating infections, it can also exacerbate autoimmune conditions by intensifying inflammatory reactions. Women with autoimmune diseases often report that their symptoms flare up during periods of hormonal change, such as menstruation, pregnancy, or menopause, suggesting a direct link between hormone levels and inflammation.

Moreover, chronic inflammation is influenced by environmental and lifestyle factors. Poor diet, stress, lack of sleep, and exposure to environmental toxins can all contribute to a state of low-grade, systemic inflammation. This persistent state of immune activation can gradually wear down the body's tolerance mechanisms, setting the stage for autoimmune reactions. In the gut, for example, a pro-inflammatory diet high in processed foods, sugar, and unhealthy fats can disrupt the gut microbiome and increase intestinal permeability, further fueling inflammation.

The dual nature of inflammation—as both a healer and a potential destroyer—underscores the importance of managing it effectively, particularly for women with autoimmune conditions. The Autoimmune Protocol (AIP) diet is designed to mitigate chronic inflammation by removing common dietary triggers and focusing on nutrient-dense foods that support immune balance. By addressing the factors that convert inflammation from a helpful response into a harmful force, women can take proactive steps to reduce symptoms and restore health.

Chapter 3:
The Gut-Immune Connection

Recent research has uncovered a powerful link between gut health and the immune system, revealing that the gut is not merely a site for digestion but also a central hub for immune regulation. Housing nearly 70% of the body's immune cells, the gastrointestinal tract plays a critical role in maintaining the delicate balance between immune tolerance and activation. For women, this connection is especially relevant, as hormonal fluctuations can impact gut function and, in turn, influence immune responses. When the gut's integrity is compromised—often due to diet, stress, or environmental toxins—its ability to act as a barrier weakens, allowing harmful substances to enter the bloodstream. This triggers a cascade of immune activity, contributing to chronic inflammation and the onset of autoimmune diseases. This chapter delves into the science of the gut-immune axis, exploring how the Autoimmune Protocol (AIP) diet can help restore gut health and, subsequently, support immune balance.

GUT HEALTH AS THE FOUNDATION OF IMMUNITY

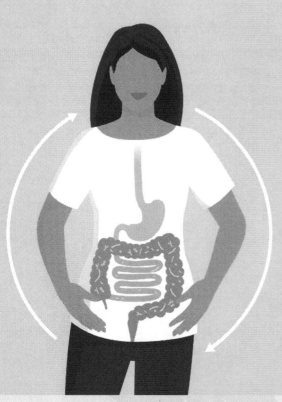

The gut is often called the "second brain," but its role extends far beyond digestion and neurological functions. It serves as the command center for much of the body's immune activity, forming the foundation of our immune defenses. The gastrointestinal (GI) tract contains a complex network of immune cells, signaling molecules, and beneficial microbes that work together to maintain a balanced state of immune vigilance. When this intricate system is functioning properly, the gut can distinguish between harmful pathogens and harmless substances, such as food particles and beneficial bacteria, allowing the immune system to respond appropriately.

The gut lining is the first line of defense in this system. Comprised of a single layer of tightly connected epithelial cells, this lining acts as a selective barrier, allowing essential nutrients to pass into the bloodstream while blocking harmful pathogens and toxins. A layer of mucus, rich in antimicrobial peptides and immunoglobulins like IgA, further strengthens this barrier, preventing unwanted substances from crossing into the body's internal environment.

However, this barrier is not static; it is highly dynamic and responsive to both internal and external cues. Dietary factors play a significant role in maintaining the integrity of the gut lining. Fiber-rich foods, for instance, promote the growth of beneficial gut bacteria that produce short-chain fatty acids (SCFAs). SCFAs, such as butyrate, help nourish the epithelial cells and maintain tight junctions—protein structures that control the permeability of the gut lining. This process is vital for preventing "leaky gut," a condition where increased intestinal permeability allows foreign particles to enter the bloodstream, potentially triggering an immune response.

The gut microbiome—a diverse community of trillions of microbes residing in the intestines—also plays a crucial role in immune regulation. These microbes interact with immune cells in the gut-associated lymphoid tissue (GALT), shaping the body's immune responses. Beneficial bacteria produce metabolites that support the development and function of regulatory T-cells (Tregs), which are essential for maintaining immune tolerance and preventing the immune system from attacking the body's own tissues. When the balance of gut bacteria is disrupted, known as dysbiosis, this regulatory function weakens, increasing the risk of chronic inflammation and autoimmunity.

For women, hormonal fluctuations can further impact gut health and, consequently, immune function. Estrogen, for example, influences the composition of the gut microbiome and affects the production of mucus that protects the gut lining. During hormonal shifts—such as during menstruation, pregnancy, or menopause—the gut environment can change, altering immune regulation. This highlights why women with autoimmune diseases often experience symptom flare-ups in sync with hormonal cycles.

Understanding that the gut is the foundation of immune health provides a clear path to intervention. The Autoimmune Protocol (AIP) diet focuses on restoring gut integrity by eliminating foods that may disrupt the gut lining, promoting the growth of beneficial bacteria, and supporting the body's natural ability to maintain immune balance. By nourishing the gut, women can take proactive steps to enhance their immunity and manage autoimmune conditions more effectively.

LEAKY GUT SYNDROME AND ITS ROLE IN AUTOIMMUNITY

Leaky gut syndrome, scientifically known as increased intestinal permeability, has emerged as a key factor in the development and exacerbation of autoimmune diseases. The term "leaky gut" refers to a condition where the normally tight junctions between the cells lining the intestinal wall become loosened or damaged. This weakening allows larger molecules—such as undigested food particles, toxins, and bacteria—to pass through the gut barrier and enter the bloodstream, an occurrence that triggers a cascade of immune reactions.

Under normal circumstances, the gut lining acts as a selective barrier, ensuring that only properly digested nutrients pass into the bloodstream while keeping harmful substances out. However, when this barrier is compromised, these unwanted particles can infiltrate the body's internal environment. The immune system, always on the lookout for potential threats, recognizes these foreign substances as invaders and mounts an inflammatory response. Over time, repeated exposure to these particles can lead to chronic immune activation, laying the groundwork for autoimmunity.

In women, several factors can contribute to the development of leaky gut syndrome. Dietary choices, such as the consumption of gluten, alcohol, and processed foods, have been shown to directly affect the tight junctions in the gut lining. Gluten, in particular, can increase the production of zonulin, a protein that regulates the permeability of the intestinal wall. Elevated levels of zonulin are associated with the loosening of tight junctions, which can create openings in the gut barrier. This is especially relevant for women with genetic predispositions to gluten sensitivity or celiac disease, as they may experience a more pronounced effect on gut integrity.

Hormonal fluctuations also play a role in modulating gut permeability. Estrogen and progesterone, hormones that fluctuate during the menstrual cycle, pregnancy, and menopause, can influence the gut lining's strength and resilience. For example, during the luteal phase of the menstrual cycle, elevated progesterone levels can alter gut motility and mucus production, potentially increasing susceptibility to gut barrier disruption. This hormonal impact may explain why some women

experience worsening autoimmune symptoms during certain times in their cycle.

Another contributing factor to leaky gut in women is chronic stress. Stress has been shown to affect gut health by increasing the release of cortisol, a hormone that can alter gut microbiota composition and reduce the production of protective mucus in the intestines. Reduced mucus can expose the epithelial cells of the gut lining to potential damage, further increasing the risk of permeability. Stress also impacts the nervous system's regulation of the gut, known as the gut-brain axis, which can exacerbate inflammation and immune dysregulation.

Once the gut becomes "leaky," the immune system is continually bombarded with foreign substances, leading to the production of autoantibodies—antibodies that mistakenly target the body's own tissues. This ongoing immune activation can contribute to the development of various autoimmune diseases, such as lupus, rheumatoid arthritis, and Hashimoto's thyroiditis. Over time, this self-attack creates a cycle of inflammation and tissue damage, intensifying autoimmune symptoms.

Addressing leaky gut is therefore a critical step in managing autoimmunity. The Autoimmune Protocol (AIP) diet specifically targets this issue by eliminating foods known to irritate the gut lining and contribute to increased permeability, while emphasizing nutrient-rich foods that support gut healing. By promoting a balanced microbiome, reducing inflammation, and restoring the gut barrier's integrity, the AIP diet provides women with an evidence-based approach to disrupting the cycle of leaky gut and autoimmunity, paving the way for symptom relief and improved health.

RECOGNIZING SIGNS OF GUT IMBALANCE

Gut imbalance, often termed dysbiosis, can be a silent contributor to many health issues, particularly autoimmune conditions. For women, understanding the signs of a gut in distress is crucial, as they can manifest in ways that may not immediately suggest digestive trouble. Recognizing these signs early can offer a pathway to intervention, allowing for dietary and lifestyle adjustments that promote gut health and, subsequently, immune balance.

One of the most common signs of gut imbalance is digestive discomfort. This can include symptoms such as bloating, gas, constipation, diarrhea, or frequent indigestion. These issues often arise when the balance of beneficial to harmful bacteria in the gut is disrupted, impairing proper digestion and nutrient absorption. For example, an overgrowth of certain bacteria can lead to excessive fermentation in the intestines, resulting in gas and bloating. On the other hand, low levels of beneficial bacteria can slow bowel movements, leading to constipation.

However, gut imbalance does not solely present as digestive distress. For many women, the signs can be more systemic and may include unexplained fatigue, joint pain, or skin issues like acne, eczema, or rashes. When the gut is out of balance, its ability to properly process and absorb essential nutrients, such as iron, vitamin D, and B vitamins, is compromised. This nutrient deficiency can lead to fatigue, decreased mental clarity, and mood disturbances. Similarly, when the gut barrier becomes more permeable, it allows inflammatory compounds to enter the bloodstream, which can trigger systemic inflammation, resulting in joint pain and skin flare-ups.

Another key sign of gut imbalance is food sensitivities or intolerances. Women with dysbiosis often notice that certain foods trigger digestive symptoms, skin reactions, or other discomforts shortly after consumption. These sensitivities occur because an imbalanced gut microbiome can weaken the gut lining, making it easier for undigested food particles to cross into the bloodstream and provoke an immune response. As the immune system becomes hyper-alert to these foreign particles, it can develop sensitivities to foods that were previously well-tolerated, leading to symptoms such as headaches, rashes, or gastrointestinal distress.

Hormonal imbalances can also be a telling sign of gut health issues, particularly for women. The gut microbiome plays a role in the metabolism and regulation of hormones, including estrogen. An imbalanced gut can impair the body's ability to properly excrete excess estrogen, resulting in symptoms like irregular menstrual cycles, severe PMS, mood swings, and even conditions such as polycystic ovary syndrome (PCOS). Recognizing the link between gut health and hormonal balance is key for women, as addressing gut issues can often help alleviate related hormonal symptoms.

Mental health symptoms, such as anxiety and depression, may also indicate gut imbalance. The gut-brain axis is a bidirectional communication system between the gut and the brain, and the state of the gut microbiome can directly impact mental health. When the gut is imbalanced, the production of neurotransmitters like serotonin—a chemical that regulates mood, sleep, and appetite—can be affected. This imbalance can contribute to feelings of anxiety, low mood, and poor stress resilience.

Being attuned to these diverse symptoms—whether they manifest as digestive disturbances, skin issues, food sensitivities, hormonal imbalances, or mental health concerns—can help women recognize when their gut might be out of balance. By acknowledging these signs, women can take proactive steps to restore gut health through interventions like the Autoimmune Protocol (AIP) diet, which aims to rebalance the microbiome, support the gut barrier, and promote overall well-being. Understanding and addressing gut imbalance is a powerful step toward managing autoimmune conditions and achieving lasting health.

Chapter 4:
Introduction to the Autoimmune Protocol (AIP) Diet

The Autoimmune Protocol (AIP) diet is more than just a meal plan—it's a strategic, science-backed approach designed to address the root causes of autoimmune conditions. Unlike other dietary strategies, AIP focuses on reducing inflammation, repairing the gut lining, and regulating immune function by eliminating foods that can trigger immune reactions. For women with autoimmune diseases, AIP offers a structured pathway to identify personal food sensitivities and to incorporate nutrient-dense options that support healing. This diet is grounded in research showing the powerful connection between diet, gut health, and immune regulation. By removing potential irritants such as gluten, dairy, grains, and processed foods while emphasizing nutrient-rich foods, the AIP diet aims to restore balance and alleviate symptoms. This chapter provides an overview of the core principles of AIP, its goals, and how it can become a transformative tool in managing autoimmune conditions and improving overall well-being.

ORIGINS AND EVOLUTION OF THE AIP DIET

The Autoimmune Protocol (AIP) diet evolved from the foundational principles of the Paleo diet, which emphasizes whole, unprocessed foods that our ancestors consumed during the Paleolithic era. The Paleo diet was originally designed to align with the human body's genetic makeup, reducing the intake of modern, processed foods that have been linked to various health issues. However, as researchers and practitioners delved deeper into the needs of individuals with autoimmune diseases, it became evident that a more targeted dietary approach was necessary. This realization gave rise to the AIP diet, tailored specifically to address the unique challenges of autoimmunity.

The AIP diet was initially developed by Dr. Loren Cordain, a pioneer in Paleo nutrition, and was later refined by researchers and practitioners like Dr. Sarah Ballantyne, who further explored the relationship between food, gut health, and the immune system. This evolving dietary approach draws from scientific research on nutritional immunology, gut microbiome dynamics, and the impacts of dietary components on inflammation and immune function. Unlike the broader Paleo diet, the AIP diet takes a more restrictive approach in its elimination phase, removing not just grains, dairy, and processed sugars, but also foods like nuts, seeds, nightshades, and eggs, which have been identified as potential immune triggers in those with autoimmune conditions.

The origins of the AIP diet are deeply rooted in the understanding that gut health is pivotal in the regulation of immune responses. Early research in autoimmunity pointed to the role of increased intestinal permeability, or "leaky gut," in the progression of autoimmune diseases. The AIP diet evolved to prioritize gut healing through the removal of foods known to disrupt the intestinal barrier. Furthermore, it emphasizes the inclusion of nutrient-dense foods—such as organ meats, leafy greens, and bone broth—that provide essential vitamins, minerals, and compounds that support immune modulation and tissue repair.

As the diet continued to evolve, practitioners recognized the importance of not just food elimination, but also systematic reintroduction of foods to identify individual triggers. This step added a personalized aspect to the protocol, allowing women to understand which foods specifically provoke their symptoms. Today, the AIP diet has gained recognition within the functional medicine community as a comprehensive lifestyle approach, incorporating not only dietary changes but also stress management, sleep optimization, and exercise to create a holistic environment for healing.

The evolution of the AIP diet reflects the growing body of scientific evidence linking dietary choices to immune regulation. It has shifted from simply being a restrictive diet to a dynamic, research-informed strategy for restoring balance within the body. By focusing on the elimination of potential irritants, the nourishment of the gut microbiome, and the individualized reintroduction of foods, the AIP diet provides a pathway for women with autoimmune conditions to regain control over their health and well-being.

THE SCIENCE SUPPORTING AIP: AN OVERVIEW OF RESEARCH

The Autoimmune Protocol (AIP) diet is grounded in a growing body of scientific research that connects diet, gut health, and immune regulation. For women grappling with autoimmune diseases, AIP offers a science-backed approach that targets the root causes of inflammation and immune dysregulation. While clinical studies on the AIP diet are still in their early stages, the research available provides compelling evidence for its efficacy in managing symptoms and improving quality of life.

One of the most notable studies on AIP was conducted in 2017, focusing on patients with inflammatory bowel disease (IBD). The study, published in the Inflammatory Bowel Diseases Journal, involved participants following the AIP diet for six weeks. Results showed a significant improvement in clinical symptoms, with 73% of participants achieving clinical remission by the end of the study. This improvement was linked to changes in dietary intake that supported gut health and reduced immune activation. The researchers concluded that dietary intervention through the AIP diet could serve as an effective adjunct therapy for managing autoimmune conditions like IBD.

Further research has explored the impact of diet on gut microbiome composition and its role in autoimmunity. Studies have found that a nutrient-rich diet, such as the one promoted by AIP, enhances the diversity and balance of gut bacteria, leading to a more regulated immune response. The AIP diet eliminates common gut irritants, such as gluten, grains, and dairy, which have been associated with increased intestinal permeability—a key factor in the development of autoimmune diseases. By promoting the consumption of foods like fermented vegetables, bone broth, and leafy greens, AIP supports the growth of beneficial gut bacteria that produce short-chain fatty acids, compounds known to strengthen the gut barrier and reduce inflammation.

A 2019 pilot study published in the Cureus Journal examined the effects of the AIP diet on women with Hashimoto's thyroiditis, an autoimmune disorder affecting the thyroid gland. Over ten weeks, participants followed a structured AIP diet plan, and results showed a significant reduction in symptoms, including fatigue, joint pain, and mental fog. The participants also experienced an average 29% decrease in markers of inflammation, suggesting that dietary modifications can have a measurable impact on autoimmune disease activity.

Additionally, research has highlighted the link between food sensitivities and autoimmune conditions. The AIP diet's elimination phase addresses this by removing foods known to trigger immune reactions in sensitive individuals. When certain proteins from foods cross the gut barrier in a leaky gut scenario, they can provoke an immune response, leading to systemic inflammation and symptom flare-ups. The structured reintroduction phase of AIP allows for the identification of specific food triggers, offering a personalized approach to autoimmune management.

Though direct clinical research on AIP is still expanding, its foundation is supported by a wide array of studies on related topics, including dietary patterns, gut health, and inflammation. The principles of AIP align with evidence that a diet low in processed foods and high in nutrient density can modulate the immune system, support gut barrier integrity, and decrease autoimmune activity. This emerging research landscape underscores AIP as a promising strategy for women seeking to alleviate symptoms and regain control of their health.

In sum, the AIP diet is not merely a restrictive eating plan but a research-supported approach that addresses the complexities of autoimmunity. By focusing on gut health, nutrient density, and the elimination of immune-triggering foods, the AIP diet is positioned as a powerful tool for improving quality of life for women with autoimmune conditions. As research continues to unfold, the AIP diet's role in autoimmunity management is likely to gain even more scientific validation.

HOW AIP DIFFERS FROM OTHER DIETS

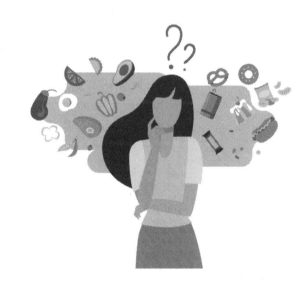

The Autoimmune Protocol (AIP) diet stands apart from other dietary approaches due to its targeted focus on managing autoimmune conditions through gut healing, immune regulation, and nutrient density. While many diets aim for general health, weight loss, or metabolic improvements, AIP is uniquely designed to address the underlying mechanisms of autoimmunity, making it a valuable option for women dealing with these complex conditions. Its comprehensive framework extends beyond mere food selection to include lifestyle factors such as stress management, sleep quality, and physical activity, all of which play critical roles in autoimmune health.

Unlike the Paleo diet, from which it originated, AIP takes a more restrictive and systematic approach by eliminating additional foods that can potentially provoke an immune response. While Paleo emphasizes whole, unprocessed foods—removing grains, dairy, legumes, and refined sugars—AIP goes further by excluding eggs, nuts, seeds, nightshade vegetables, and food additives. This added layer of restriction is based on research indicating that certain compounds in these foods, such as saponins in nightshades and lectins in legumes, can increase gut permeability and trigger inflammation in those with autoimmune diseases.

A key difference between AIP and gluten-free or dairy-free diets is that AIP is not limited to the exclusion of one specific group of foods. Although gluten and dairy are both removed in AIP due to their potential to disrupt the gut lining and trigger immune reactions, the diet also targets other common inflammatory foods. The aim is to reduce the overall immune load, giving the body an opportunity to reset and heal. This comprehensive elimination phase, followed by a structured reintroduction process, allows women to identify their specific dietary triggers, which is not the focus of conventional gluten-free or dairy-free plans.

Similarly, while low FODMAP diets are often used to manage gastrointestinal symptoms, particularly in conditions like irritable bowel syndrome (IBS), they do not address the broader immune and inflammatory aspects that AIP targets. Low FODMAP diets primarily focus on reducing fermentable carbohydrates that can cause bloating, gas, and discomfort. In contrast, AIP's goal is to restore gut integrity and balance the immune system by eliminating foods that contribute to chronic inflammation, supporting both digestive health and immune modulation.

Another diet often compared to AIP is the Mediterranean diet, which emphasizes whole grains, legumes, lean proteins, healthy fats, and ample fruits and vegetables. While rich in anti-inflammatory foods like olive oil, fish, and leafy greens, the Mediterranean diet includes grains and legumes—both of which are eliminated in the AIP diet due to their potential to provoke immune reactions and exacerbate intestinal permeability in individuals with autoimmune conditions. AIP's approach is more targeted, removing foods that might impair the gut lining, which is essential for individuals who experience autoimmune symptoms.

AIP also differs significantly from ketogenic diets, which focus on drastically reducing carbohydrate intake to shift the body into a state of ketosis, where fat becomes the primary fuel source. While keto can have anti-inflammatory benefits for some individuals, it does not prioritize the elimination of foods that may trigger autoimmune responses, such as dairy, eggs, and certain nuts. AIP emphasizes gut health and immune regulation rather than macronutrient composition, making it more suitable for women dealing with autoimmune conditions who may not benefit from extreme carb restriction.

One of the most defining aspects of AIP is its systematic reintroduction phase, which sets it apart from other elimination diets. After a period of eliminating potential inflammatory foods, AIP encourages careful, one-at-a-time reintroduction to identify specific food triggers. This process provides a personalized blueprint for long-term dietary choices, allowing women to customize their diet based on their body's unique responses. Unlike other diets that may focus on universal restrictions, AIP's individualized approach recognizes that autoimmune conditions vary from person to person, necessitating a tailored strategy.

In summary, AIP differs from other diets in its comprehensive elimination phase, focus on nutrient density, and attention to gut and immune health. It goes beyond basic dietary adjustments to include lifestyle changes that support healing and provide a more holistic solution for managing autoimmune diseases. For women, this approach offers a science-backed pathway to identify and eliminate their specific triggers, restore gut balance, and modulate immune function, leading to a better quality of life.

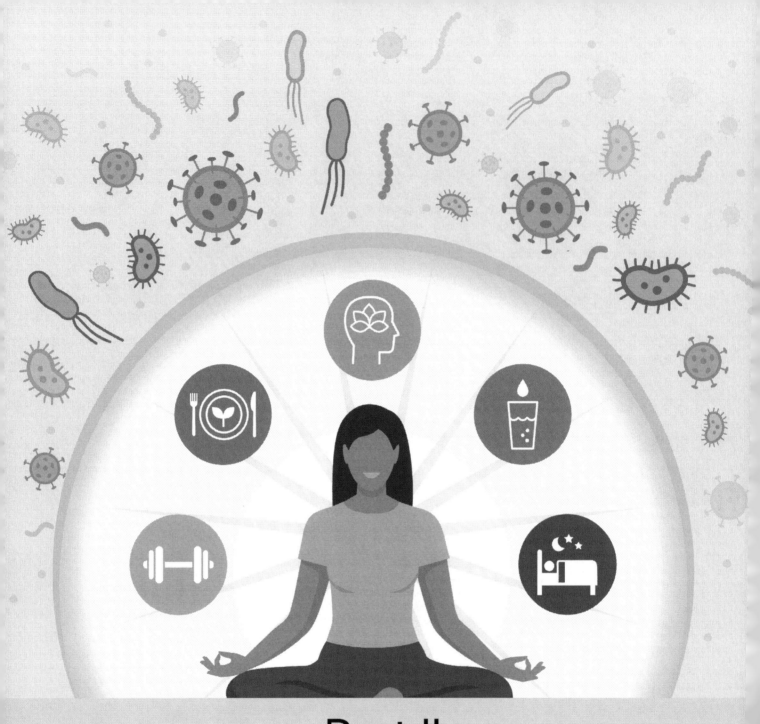

Part II:
The 7 Essential Pillars to Restore Your Immune System

Chapter 5:
Pillar 1 – The Elimination Phase

The Elimination Phase is the cornerstone of the Autoimmune Protocol (AIP) diet, designed to remove foods that may trigger immune reactions, increase inflammation, and disrupt gut health. This phase requires a highly targeted approach, temporarily excluding foods known to provoke adverse reactions in individuals with autoimmune conditions. Unlike traditional restrictive diets, the AIP Elimination Phase focuses on identifying specific dietary triggers, setting the stage for gut healing and immune regulation. For women, this process can be particularly impactful, as hormonal fluctuations and lifestyle factors can exacerbate immune sensitivity. By eliminating foods such as grains, dairy, legumes, nightshades, eggs, nuts, seeds, and food additives, the body is given a chance to reset and repair the gut lining. This chapter outlines the scientific rationale behind the elimination of these foods and provides practical guidance on how to navigate this crucial phase to support symptom relief and long-term wellness.

UNDERSTANDING FOOD TRIGGERS AND SENSITIVITIES

In autoimmune diseases, food triggers and sensitivities can act as silent culprits, exacerbating symptoms and fueling inflammation. Unlike food allergies, which elicit an immediate and sometimes severe immune response, food sensitivities produce delayed reactions that can be more challenging to identify. These reactions occur when the immune system recognizes certain food components—such as proteins, additives, or naturally occurring compounds—as threats, resulting in chronic, low-grade inflammation. For women, understanding and addressing these food triggers is crucial, as they can directly influence not only digestive health but also hormonal balance, energy levels, and immune function.

One of the most common food triggers in autoimmune conditions is gluten, a protein found in wheat, rye, and barley. Gluten has been shown to increase intestinal permeability, particularly in individuals with genetic predispositions such as celiac disease and non-celiac gluten sensitivity. This increased permeability, often referred to as "leaky gut," allows undigested food particles and toxins to cross into the bloodstream, activating the immune system and contributing to the onset and progression of autoimmune reactions. For many women, consuming gluten can result in a range of symptoms, from digestive discomfort to joint pain and brain fog, making its elimination during the AIP diet's initial phase essential for gut healing.

Dairy products, another common trigger, contain proteins like casein and whey, which can be difficult for some people to digest. In sensitive individuals, dairy consumption can provoke an immune response, leading to inflammation and exacerbating symptoms such as bloating, skin rashes, or joint pain. Additionally, dairy can affect the hormonal axis in women, as it contains bioactive hormones and growth factors that can interfere with the body's natural hormone regulation. For this reason, the AIP diet eliminates dairy in its entirety during the Elimination Phase to assess its impact on individual symptoms.

Nightshade vegetables—including tomatoes, peppers, eggplants, and potatoes—contain compounds like alkaloids, saponins, and lectins, which can be problematic for those with autoimmune diseases. These compounds have the potential to irritate the gut lining and provoke immune responses, particularly in individuals with already heightened immune sensitivity. Nightshades can also influence joint pain, a common symptom in conditions like rheumatoid arthritis, by promoting inflammatory pathways within the body.

Nuts and seeds are typically regarded as healthful foods due to their nutrient density, but they can act as triggers for some women with autoimmunity. They contain phytic acid and lectins, which may impair nutrient absorption and aggravate the gut lining. Additionally, their high omega-6 fatty acid content can contribute to an imbalance in the body's omega-3 to omega-6 ratio, potentially promoting inflammation. Therefore, nuts and seeds are removed during the Elimination Phase to gauge their effects on immune function and inflammation.

Eggs, a common breakfast staple, are also excluded during the Elimination Phase. The proteins in egg whites, particularly albumin, can be difficult for some individuals to digest, potentially provoking an immune response. Furthermore, the yolk contains arachidonic acid, which is a precursor to pro-inflammatory molecules in the body. For women experiencing autoimmune symptoms, removing eggs allows the gut to heal and reduces the burden on the immune system.

In addition to these common triggers, food additives such as emulsifiers, artificial sweeteners, and preservatives can disrupt gut microbiota balance and increase intestinal permeability, further aggravating immune responses. This highlights the importance of eliminating not only natural foods that may cause sensitivities but also processed foods that contain harmful additives.

Understanding food triggers is key to the success of the AIP diet. The systematic removal of these potential irritants provides the body an opportunity to reset, reducing inflammation and calming the immune system. This Elimination Phase is not about permanently banning foods but about discovering which specific foods your body reacts to. Through this process, women can develop a personalized dietary blueprint that minimizes symptoms, supports gut health, and promotes overall immune balance.

COMPREHENSIVE LIST OF FOODS TO ELIMINATE

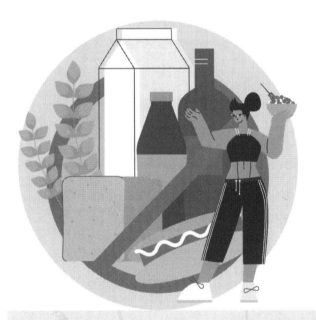

The Elimination Phase of the Autoimmune Protocol (AIP) diet is a targeted approach to identify and remove foods that may contribute to inflammation, gut permeability, and immune dysregulation. This phase involves eliminating specific food groups known for their potential to provoke immune reactions, irritate the gut lining, or disrupt the body's natural balance. By temporarily excluding these foods, women with autoimmune conditions can create an optimal environment for healing and immune modulation. Below is a detailed, science-backed list of the foods to be eliminated during this phase.

1. Grains

Grains contain compounds such as gluten, lectins, and phytic acid, which can increase intestinal permeability and trigger immune responses, particularly in those with a genetic predisposition to autoimmunity. All grains, including:

- Gluten-containing grains: Wheat, barley, rye, spelt, and products made from these grains like bread, pasta, and cereal.

- Gluten-free grains: Rice, oats, corn, quinoa, millet, and buckwheat.

2. Legumes

Legumes contain lectins and saponins that may irritate the gut lining, as well as phytic acid, which can bind minerals and inhibit nutrient absorption. During the Elimination Phase, avoid:

- All beans: Kidney beans, black beans, navy beans, pinto beans, lentils, chickpeas, and soybeans.

- Soy products: Tofu, tempeh, soy milk, and edamame.

- Peanuts and peanut butter (as they are technically legumes, not nuts).

3. Dairy

Dairy products contain proteins like casein and lactose, which can be difficult to digest and may provoke inflammatory responses. Additionally, dairy can interfere with hormonal balance. The AIP diet eliminates all forms of dairy, including:

- Milk and milk products: Cow's milk, goat's milk, cheese, yogurt, kefir, cream, and butter.

- Ghee: While often considered a dairy-free alternative, ghee still contains trace amounts of milk proteins that can affect sensitive individuals.

4. Nightshade Vegetables

Nightshades contain alkaloids and lectins that can irritate the gut lining and potentially trigger inflammatory pathways. Common nightshades to exclude:

- Vegetables: Tomatoes, potatoes (excluding sweet potatoes), eggplants, peppers (bell peppers, chili peppers, jalapeños, etc.).

- Spices derived from nightshades: Paprika, cayenne pepper, chili powder, and curry powders containing these ingredients.

5. Nuts and Seeds

Nuts and seeds are nutrient-dense but can contain phytic acid and lectins that interfere with digestion and nutrient absorption. They also have a high omega-6 fatty acid content, which can contribute to inflammation. During this phase, eliminate:

- All nuts: Almonds, walnuts, pecans, cashews, pistachios, macadamia nuts, and hazelnuts.

- All seeds: Chia seeds, flaxseeds, pumpkin seeds, sunflower seeds, sesame seeds.

- Nut and seed-derived products: Nut butters (almond butter, cashew butter), nut milks (almond milk, cashew milk), seed oils (sesame oil, sunflower oil).

6. Eggs

Eggs, particularly the egg whites, contain proteins like albumin that can trigger immune responses and contribute to inflammation. For women experiencing autoimmune symptoms, removing eggs during this phase is essential. Avoid:

- Whole eggs: Including both whites and yolks.

- Products containing eggs: Baked goods, mayonnaise, and certain condiments.

7. Processed Foods and Additives

Processed foods often contain artificial additives, preservatives, emulsifiers, and refined sugars that can disrupt gut microbiota balance and exacerbate inflammation. Eliminate:

- Packaged snacks: Chips, cookies, crackers, and energy bars.

- Processed meats: Sausages, hot dogs, deli meats, bacon, and canned meats.

- Artificial sweeteners: Aspartame, sucralose, saccharin, and stevia.

- Food additives: Emulsifiers (like polysorbate 80), carrageenan, guar gum, xanthan gum, and food colorings.

8. Refined Sugars and Sweeteners

Refined sugars can contribute to blood sugar imbalances and promote inflammation. During the Elimination Phase, avoid:

- Refined sugars: White sugar, brown sugar, cane sugar, high-fructose corn syrup.

- Artificial sweeteners: Sucralose, aspartame, saccharin.

- Natural sweeteners: While honey and maple syrup are generally allowed in moderation, it's best to avoid all sweeteners during the initial phase to assess their impact.

9. Alcohol and Caffeine

Both alcohol and caffeine can disrupt gut integrity, alter hormone levels, and increase stress on the immune system. For optimal results during the Elimination Phase:

- Avoid all forms of alcohol: Wine, beer, spirits, and cocktails.

- Avoid caffeine: Coffee, black tea, green tea, and caffeinated sodas.

10. Certain Oils and Fats

Processed vegetable oils are high in omega-6 fatty acids, which can promote an inflammatory response when consumed in excess. During this phase, eliminate:

- Processed oils: Canola oil, soybean oil, corn oil, sunflower oil, and safflower oil.

- Margarine and hydrogenated oils: Often found in processed foods and baked goods.

This comprehensive elimination allows the immune system to reset and the gut lining to heal. Remember, the goal is not lifelong exclusion but a temporary period to help identify which foods are safe to reintroduce in the later stages of the AIP diet. By committing to this process, women can gain clarity on their individual food triggers and tailor their diets to support their unique autoimmune needs.

Chapter 6:
Pillar 2 – Embracing Nutrient-Dense Foods

Nutrient density is at the heart of the Autoimmune Protocol (AIP) diet, focusing on foods rich in essential vitamins, minerals, antioxidants, and phytonutrients that support immune health, reduce inflammation, and promote gut healing. For women with autoimmune conditions, embracing nutrient-dense foods is crucial to fill the nutritional gaps often caused by restricted diets, compromised digestion, or chronic inflammation. Unlike traditional diets that simply limit calories or certain macronutrients, AIP prioritizes the quality and diversity of nutrients. Foods like leafy greens, organ meats, bone broth, and fermented vegetables are included to provide a broad spectrum of nutrients, including iron, zinc, magnesium, omega-3 fatty acids, and vitamins A, D, E, and K. This chapter explores the scientific rationale behind the inclusion of these nutrient-dense foods, explaining how they can restore balance to the body, support hormone regulation, and strengthen the immune system, setting the foundation for long-term wellness.

THE IMPORTANCE OF MICRONUTRIENTS IN HEALING

Micronutrients, including vitamins and minerals, are the unsung heroes of the healing process, especially in the context of autoimmune conditions. While they are required in small amounts, their impact on immune function, cellular repair, and overall health is profound. For women dealing with autoimmunity, ensuring an adequate intake of these vital nutrients is crucial, as deficiencies can exacerbate symptoms, impair immune regulation, and slow down the body's natural healing mechanisms.

Vitamins, such as A, D, E, and K, play a pivotal role in modulating the immune response. Vitamin A, for instance, is essential for maintaining the integrity of the gut lining, a key barrier against harmful pathogens and toxins. It also supports the production and activity of T-cells, which are crucial for distinguishing between harmful invaders and the body's own tissues. Inadequate levels of vitamin A can compromise these immune functions, potentially worsening autoimmune flare-ups.

Vitamin D, often referred to as the "sunshine vitamin," is especially important for women with autoimmune conditions. Research shows that vitamin D helps regulate the immune system, promoting tolerance and preventing it from mistakenly attacking healthy tissues. It plays a role in the production of regulatory T-cells (Tregs), which suppress excessive inflammatory responses. Vitamin D deficiencies are common among individuals with autoimmune diseases, and addressing this deficiency can significantly improve symptom management and immune balance.

Minerals, such as zinc, magnesium, selenium, and iron, are equally critical for immune health and cellular repair. Zinc, for example, is essential for the proper function of immune cells, including natural killer (NK) cells and T-cells. It also plays a role in maintaining the integrity of the epithelial barriers, such as the gut lining, thereby preventing the entry of potential immune triggers into the bloodstream. For women, zinc is also involved in hormone synthesis, which can help balance the hormonal fluctuations that often exacerbate autoimmune symptoms.

Magnesium is another key mineral that impacts both the immune system and overall well-being. It participates in over 300 enzymatic reactions in the body, including those involved in inflammatory regulation. Magnesium has been shown to reduce the production of pro-inflammatory cytokines, thereby helping to mitigate chronic inflammation associated with autoimmune conditions. Low magnesium levels are linked to increased stress and poor sleep, both of which can further disrupt immune function and trigger symptom flare-ups.

Iron, crucial for the production of hemoglobin and oxygen transport in the blood, is often depleted in individuals with autoimmune diseases, particularly women. Conditions like Hashimoto's thyroiditis and rheumatoid arthritis are frequently associated with anemia, as chronic inflammation can interfere with iron absorption and utilization. Including iron-rich, nutrient-dense foods such as organ meats and leafy greens in the diet can help replenish iron stores, boost energy levels, and support the body's natural healing processes.

Selenium, a powerful antioxidant, plays a protective role in reducing oxidative stress, a known contributor to autoimmune flare-ups. It is particularly important for thyroid health, as selenium is required for the conversion of the thyroid hormone T4 into its active form, T3. Adequate selenium intake has been associated with improved thyroid function and a reduction in autoimmune thyroid symptoms, making it an essential micronutrient for women with conditions like Hashimoto's thyroiditis.

Beyond these specific vitamins and minerals, the AIP diet also emphasizes foods rich in phytonutrients—bioactive compounds found in plant foods that offer additional immune-supportive and anti-inflammatory benefits. Polyphenols in fruits and vegetables, for example, have been shown to positively modulate gut microbiota composition, supporting a balanced immune response.

Ensuring a diet rich in micronutrients is, therefore, a cornerstone of the AIP diet's healing philosophy. By embracing nutrient-dense foods like leafy greens, organ meats, fatty fish, bone broth, and fermented vegetables, women can supply their bodies with the essential vitamins and minerals needed to promote immune regulation, reduce inflammation, and support cellular repair. This micronutrient-focused approach helps address potential deficiencies and provides the body with the tools it needs to recover from the effects of autoimmunity, laying the foundation for long-term health and resilience.

TOP NUTRIENT-RICH FOODS TO INCLUDE

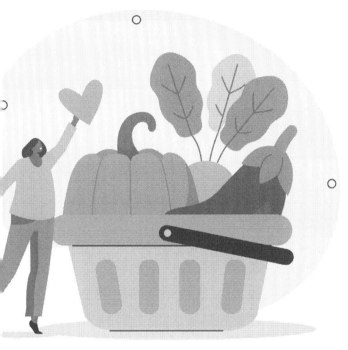

Incorporating nutrient-dense foods into your daily diet is essential for managing autoimmune conditions and promoting overall wellness. These foods are specifically chosen for their high concentrations of vitamins, minerals, antioxidants, and healthy fats, all of which play a critical role in supporting the immune system, reducing inflammation, and aiding tissue repair. For women dealing with the complexities of autoimmunity, focusing on nutrient-dense options ensures that the body receives the necessary building blocks to support hormonal balance, energy production, and gut health. Here's a comprehensive look at some of the top nutrient-rich foods to include during the AIP diet.

1. Organ Meats

Organ meats, such as liver, heart, and kidneys, are among the most nutrient-dense foods available. Liver, in particular, is an excellent source of vitamin A, iron, zinc, and B vitamins, including B12 and folate. Vitamin A is

crucial for maintaining the integrity of mucosal barriers, such as the gut lining, while iron and B12 support red blood cell production and oxygen transport. Zinc from organ meats aids in immune cell function, promoting a balanced immune response. Including organ meats in your diet at least once or twice a week provides a concentrated source of these vital nutrients, especially important for women who may be at risk for anemia and hormonal imbalances.

2. Fatty Fish

Fatty fish like salmon, mackerel, sardines, and herring are rich in omega-3 fatty acids, specifically EPA (eicosapentaenoic acid) and DHA (docosahexaenoic acid). Omega-3s have been shown to possess potent anti-inflammatory properties, reducing the production of pro-inflammatory cytokines and supporting immune modulation. Women with autoimmune conditions often experience elevated inflammation levels, and including fatty fish in the diet can help rebalance this response. Additionally, fatty fish provide high-quality protein and are an excellent source of vitamin D, another critical nutrient for immune regulation.

3. Bone Broth

Bone broth is a staple in the AIP diet, known for its gut-healing properties. It is rich in collagen, gelatin, and amino acids like glutamine, which help strengthen the gut lining and promote intestinal repair. Glutamine serves as a key fuel source for the cells lining the intestines, supporting their regeneration and maintaining tight junction integrity, thereby reducing the risk of leaky gut syndrome. Bone broth also contains trace minerals, including magnesium, calcium, and phosphorus, which play a role in cellular function and overall health. Regular consumption of bone broth can aid in soothing inflammation, improving digestion, and enhancing nutrient absorption.

4. Leafy Greens and Cruciferous Vegetables

Leafy greens such as kale, spinach, Swiss chard, and arugula, as well as cruciferous vegetables like broccoli, cauliflower, and Brussels sprouts, are packed with vitamins, minerals, and phytonutrients. They are excellent sources of magnesium, calcium, folate, vitamin C, and vitamin K. Magnesium is essential for over 300 enzymatic reactions in the body, including those related to energy production and hormone balance. Vitamin K works synergistically with vitamin D to support bone health, an important consideration for women, particularly during menopause. Additionally, cruciferous vegetables contain compounds like sulforaphane, known for their anti-inflammatory and detoxifying effects, helping to mitigate autoimmune symptoms.

5. Fermented Foods

Fermented foods such as sauerkraut, kimchi, coconut yogurt, and kombucha are rich in beneficial probiotics that support a healthy gut microbiome. The balance of gut bacteria plays a key role in immune system regulation, as gut dysbiosis is often linked to increased intestinal permeability and autoimmune flare-ups. Including fermented foods in the diet introduces beneficial bacteria, which in turn produce short-chain fatty acids (SCFAs) that nourish the cells of the gut lining and reduce inflammation. For women, maintaining a balanced microbiome is also vital for hormonal regulation and improved digestion, making fermented foods a valuable addition to the AIP diet.

6. Berries and Low-Glycemic Fruits

Berries such as blueberries, raspberries, blackberries, and strawberries are nutrient powerhouses, providing high levels of antioxidants, fiber, and vitamin C. The polyphenols found in berries, like anthocyanins and flavonoids, have been shown to modulate the immune system and protect cells from oxidative stress, a common issue in autoimmune conditions. Low-glycemic fruits, including green apples, pears, and citrus fruits, offer a source of natural sugars without causing significant spikes in blood glucose levels, thereby promoting stable energy and mood—both critical factors for women managing autoimmune symptoms.

6. Healthy Fats

Healthy fats, such as those found in avocados, olive oil, coconut oil, and coconut milk, are crucial for reducing inflammation and supporting cellular health. Avocados provide a wealth of monounsaturated fats, fiber, and potassium, which help regulate blood pressure and support heart health. Olive oil, rich in oleic acid, has anti-inflammatory properties and supports the absorption of fat-soluble vitamins (A, D, E, and K), which are essential for immune function and hormone synthesis. Coconut oil and coconut milk contain medium-chain triglycerides (MCTs), which provide a readily available source of energy and support metabolic health.

7. Herbs and Spices

While many spices are avoided in the initial AIP elimination phase, herbs like rosemary, thyme, basil, and oregano are allowed and offer antioxidant and anti-inflammatory benefits. These herbs are rich in polyphenols and flavonoids, which have been shown to support immune health and combat oxidative stress. Incorporating a variety of these fresh herbs into your cooking adds both flavor and nutrients, enhancing the overall quality of your diet.

Incorporating these nutrient-rich foods into daily meals supports the body's natural healing processes, provides essential micronutrients, and helps to balance the immune system. By focusing on these powerhouse foods, women can ensure they are fueling their bodies with the nutrients needed to alleviate symptoms, restore gut health, and optimize overall wellness.

Chapter 7:
Pillar 3 – Healing the Gut

Healing the gut is a critical component of managing autoimmune conditions, as the health of the gastrointestinal tract directly influences immune function. For women with autoimmune diseases, a compromised gut—often referred to as "leaky gut"—can lead to chronic inflammation, nutrient deficiencies, and an overactive immune system. The Autoimmune Protocol (AIP) diet emphasizes not only the elimination of foods that can damage the gut lining but also the incorporation of foods and practices that actively promote gut repair. This chapter delves into the science of gut healing, highlighting how factors such as collagen-rich bone broth, probiotic foods, and prebiotic fibers contribute to the restoration of a balanced gut microbiome and a resilient intestinal barrier. By understanding the specific strategies for supporting gut health, women can reduce systemic inflammation, improve nutrient absorption, and create a foundation for long-term autoimmune management and overall well-being.

THE ROLE OF THE GUT MICROBIOME

The gut microbiome, a diverse community of trillions of microorganisms residing in the intestines, plays a central role in maintaining immune balance, gut integrity, and overall health. This complex ecosystem, comprising bacteria, viruses, fungi, and other microbes, directly influences how the body processes food, absorbs nutrients, and regulates immune responses. For women with autoimmune conditions, the composition and balance of the gut microbiome are particularly crucial, as research has shown that disruptions in this microbial environment can trigger or exacerbate autoimmune symptoms.

A healthy gut microbiome supports immune regulation by promoting the development and function of regulatory T-cells (Tregs), which help keep the immune system in check and prevent it from mistakenly attacking the body's own tissues. The microbiome produces short-chain fatty acids (SCFAs) such as butyrate, propionate, and acetate, which have anti-inflammatory properties. These SCFAs not only nourish the cells lining the intestines, enhancing the gut barrier's integrity, but also signal to the immune system to maintain a state of tolerance rather than chronic activation. This is particularly important for women, as a well-functioning microbiome can modulate the immune system's sensitivity during various hormonal phases, reducing the likelihood of autoimmune flare-ups.

However, several factors, including diet, stress, medications, and environmental toxins, can disrupt the balance of the microbiome, leading to a state of dysbiosis. Dysbiosis is characterized by an overgrowth of harmful bacteria and a reduction in beneficial species, which can compromise the gut barrier, increase intestinal permeability, and trigger immune responses. When the gut barrier becomes "leaky," toxins, undigested food particles, and bacterial fragments can pass into the bloodstream, provoking systemic inflammation and activating autoimmune pathways. Women, due to hormonal fluctuations and a generally higher prevalence of autoimmune conditions, may be more susceptible to the impacts of dysbiosis.

One aspect of the microbiome that directly affects women's health is its role in hormone metabolism. Certain gut bacteria are involved in the breakdown and recycling of hormones like estrogen, a process known as the estrobolome. An imbalance in the gut microbiome can alter estrogen levels, potentially contributing to hormonal dysregulation and increasing the risk of hormone-related conditions, including autoimmune diseases such as Hashimoto's thyroiditis and lupus. This interconnection underscores the importance of nurturing a balanced microbiome to support both immune and hormonal health.

Dietary choices significantly influence the composition of the gut microbiome. A diet rich in fiber, prebiotics, fermented foods, and healthy fats can promote the growth of beneficial microbes, thereby enhancing immune regulation and gut integrity. Conversely, processed foods, refined sugars, artificial additives, and certain medications like antibiotics and non-steroidal anti-inflammatory drugs (NSAIDs) can disrupt the microbial balance, contributing to inflammation and immune dysregulation. The AIP diet's emphasis on whole, nutrient-dense foods and the exclusion of inflammatory substances is designed to restore and support a healthy microbiome.

Including probiotic-rich foods such as sauerkraut, kimchi, coconut yogurt, and kombucha introduces beneficial bacteria into the gut, aiding in microbial diversity. Similarly, consuming prebiotic foods like garlic, onions, and asparagus provides the necessary fuel for these beneficial microbes, promoting their growth and activity. This symbiotic relationship between prebiotics and probiotics helps fortify the gut lining, reduce inflammation, and modulate immune responses, contributing to symptom relief in women with autoimmune conditions.

In summary, the gut microbiome is a key player in immune regulation, hormonal balance, and gut health.

By focusing on restoring microbial diversity and promoting a healthy microbiome through dietary and lifestyle interventions, women can address a fundamental aspect of autoimmunity, setting the stage for improved overall health and well-being.

FOODS AND SUPPLEMENTS TO REPAIR THE GUT LINING

The health of the gut lining is pivotal for regulating immune responses and preventing autoimmune flare-ups. The intestinal lining serves as a critical barrier, selectively allowing nutrients to pass into the bloodstream while blocking harmful substances like pathogens, toxins, and undigested food particles. When this barrier becomes compromised—a condition known as increased intestinal permeability or "leaky gut"—it can lead to systemic inflammation and exacerbate autoimmune symptoms. For women, who are more prone to autoimmune conditions and are often affected by hormonal fluctuations that can impact gut health, actively repairing the gut lining is essential. Incorporating specific foods and supplements can support the gut's natural healing process, restore integrity to the intestinal barrier, and promote overall immune balance.

1. Bone Broth

Bone broth is a rich source of collagen, gelatin, and amino acids like glycine and proline, all of which are crucial for repairing the gut lining. Collagen contains compounds that support the regeneration of the epithelial cells lining the intestines, helping to tighten the junctions between these cells and prevent leakage. Gelatin, derived from collagen, forms a soothing gel-like substance that coats the intestinal walls, promoting healing and reducing inflammation. Regular consumption of bone broth provides the gut with nutrients necessary for tissue repair, making it an excellent foundational food for women looking to enhance their digestive health and alleviate autoimmune symptoms.

2. Fermented Foods

Fermented foods such as sauerkraut, kimchi, coconut yogurt, and kombucha are rich in probiotics, which introduce beneficial bacteria to the gut and help restore a balanced microbiome. A diverse and healthy microbiome plays a key role in maintaining the gut lining's integrity. Probiotic bacteria produce short-chain fatty acids (SCFAs) like butyrate, which nourish the cells of the intestinal lining, promoting their growth and function. These beneficial microbes also produce protective mucus that forms an additional barrier against harmful pathogens, supporting the healing process of a compromised gut. Including fermented foods in your diet can thus bolster gut health, support immune regulation, and contribute to the repair of the gut lining.

3. Omega-3 Fatty Acids

Foods rich in omega-3 fatty acids, such as fatty fish (salmon, mackerel, sardines) and chia seeds, have potent anti-inflammatory effects that can aid in gut healing. Chronic inflammation is a key factor in gut permeability, and omega-3s have been shown to reduce the production of pro-inflammatory cytokines, thereby creating a more conducive environment for the gut lining to repair itself. Omega-3 fatty acids also support the production of mucus in the gut, which protects the epithelial cells from irritation and damage. For women, who may experience cyclical hormonal changes that can influence inflammatory pathways, maintaining a diet rich in omega-3s is beneficial for both gut and immune health.

4. L-Glutamine

L-Glutamine is an amino acid that serves as a primary fuel source for the cells of the intestinal lining, known as enterocytes. During times of stress, illness, or compromised gut health, the body's demand for glutamine increases, making supplementation particularly helpful. Research indicates that glutamine helps strengthen the tight junctions between intestinal cells, reducing permeability and promoting the regeneration of the gut lining. For women experiencing digestive distress or autoimmune flare-ups, a daily glutamine supplement can provide targeted support for gut repair. While glutamine is also found in foods like bone broth, cabbage, and spinach, supplementation offers a more concentrated dose to accelerate healing.

5. Zinc

Zinc is an essential mineral that plays a vital role in immune function and tissue repair, including the maintenance of the gut lining. Zinc supplementation has been shown to strengthen the gut barrier by promoting the production of proteins that form the tight junctions between intestinal cells. This mineral also supports the production of mucus, offering an additional layer of protection against harmful substances. Women, who may be at risk of zinc deficiency due to dietary restrictions or increased physiological demands, can benefit from incorporating zinc-rich foods such as shellfish, pumpkin seeds, and meat into their diet, or from using a high-quality zinc supplement as recommended by a healthcare professional.

6. Aloe Vera

Aloe vera, known for its soothing properties, can help reduce inflammation and promote tissue healing in the gut. The gel from aloe vera contains polysaccharides that have been shown to enhance the healing of the intestinal lining and reduce gut permeability. Additionally, aloe vera has prebiotic effects, supporting the growth of beneficial gut bacteria. Consuming aloe vera juice in small, controlled amounts can be part of a gut-healing strategy, particularly for women who may experience inflammatory bowel symptoms as part of their autoimmune condition.

7. Licorice Root (DGL)

Deglycyrrhizinated licorice (DGL) is a form of licorice root extract that has been processed to remove glycyrrhizin, which can raise blood pressure in large amounts. DGL has mucilaginous properties, meaning it forms a protective coating on the mucous membranes, including those lining the gut. This protective layer can shield the intestines from irritants, giving the cells time to repair and regenerate. DGL is available in supplement form, typically as chewable tablets, and can be beneficial for women experiencing digestive discomfort or those seeking to enhance gut repair.

8. Gelatin and Collagen Supplements

Beyond bone broth, powdered gelatin and collagen supplements offer a convenient way to support gut health. These supplements contain amino acids, such as glycine, which play a key role in repairing the gut lining by stimulating the production of connective tissue. Women can add collagen powder to smoothies, soups, or herbal teas to provide their bodies with the necessary nutrients to rebuild the gut barrier, reduce permeability, and support overall digestive health.

9. Prebiotic-Rich Foods

Prebiotics, the non-digestible fibers that feed beneficial gut bacteria, are crucial for maintaining a healthy microbiome and supporting gut integrity. Foods like garlic, onions, leeks, asparagus, and green bananas are rich in prebiotic fibers such as inulin and fructooligosaccharides. Consuming prebiotic-rich foods encourages the growth of beneficial bacteria that produce short-chain fatty acids, which in turn nourish the cells of the gut lining and enhance its repair. This prebiotic support is especially important for women, as it promotes a balanced microbiome, which is integral to both gut health and hormonal balance.

By incorporating these foods and supplements into daily routines, women can actively support the repair of their gut lining, reduce inflammation, and create a more balanced immune environment. This approach not only addresses the immediate symptoms of a leaky gut but also lays the groundwork for long-term management of autoimmune conditions and overall health improvement.

INCORPORATING PROBIOTICS AND PREBIOTICS

Probiotics and prebiotics are essential components of a balanced diet, particularly for women managing autoimmune conditions. These two elements work synergistically to support a healthy gut microbiome, which plays a critical role in regulating immune function, reducing inflammation, and maintaining the integrity of the gut lining. Incorporating both probiotics and prebiotics into daily nutrition can promote microbial diversity, enhance gut health, and contribute to a more balanced immune response.

Probiotics: Introducing Beneficial Bacteria

Probiotics are live microorganisms, primarily beneficial bacteria, that, when consumed in adequate amounts, confer health benefits to the host. The gut microbiome comprises a complex community of bacteria, and the balance between beneficial and potentially harmful species is key to maintaining overall health. Research shows that a diverse microbiome is associated with a well-regulated immune system, and probiotic supplementation can help restore microbial balance, particularly when dysbiosis (an imbalance of gut bacteria) is present.

For women, incorporating probiotics into their diet is especially important because a well-functioning microbiome can help regulate hormonal balance, support digestion, and protect against autoimmune flare-ups. Foods rich in natural probiotics include fermented products such as:

- Sauerkraut: Made from fermented cabbage, sauerkraut provides strains of Lactobacillus bacteria, which support the production of short-chain fatty acids (SCFAs) that nourish the cells of the gut lining.

- Kimchi: A Korean fermented vegetable dish that is rich in beneficial bacteria like Lactobacillus plantarum, kimchi helps modulate the immune system and reduce gut inflammation.

- Coconut Yogurt: A dairy-free alternative that contains active cultures of Lactobacillus and Bifidobacterium strains, aiding in the maintenance of a balanced gut microbiome.

- Kombucha: A fermented tea that contains beneficial yeast and bacteria, kombucha promotes digestive health and microbial diversity in the gut.

While probiotic-rich foods can be an effective way to introduce beneficial bacteria, women with specific gut health challenges may benefit from probiotic supplements. When selecting a supplement, it's important to look for products containing well-researched strains, such as Lactobacillus acidophilus, Lactobacillus rhamnosus, and Bifidobacterium lactis, which have been shown to enhance gut barrier function and modulate immune responses. Additionally, opting for a supplement with multiple strains can provide a broader spectrum of benefits for gut health.

Prebiotics: Fueling the Beneficial Bacteria

Prebiotics are non-digestible fibers that serve as food for the beneficial bacteria in the gut. Unlike probiotics, which introduce live microorganisms, prebiotics stimulate the growth and activity of the already present beneficial bacteria. They help produce SCFAs, like butyrate, which have anti-inflammatory properties and play a vital role in maintaining the integrity of the gut lining. For women, prebiotics can support a healthier microbiome, which can positively impact hormonal regulation and immune modulation.

Incorporating prebiotic-rich foods into the diet can help sustain a healthy microbial environment. Some of the best prebiotic sources include:

- Garlic: Rich in inulin, a type of prebiotic fiber, garlic supports the growth of beneficial bacteria like Bifidobacterium and Lactobacillus. It also contains antimicrobial properties that can help regulate the growth of harmful gut bacteria.

- Onions and Leeks: High in fructooligosaccharides (FOS), onions and leeks provide fuel for beneficial bacteria, promoting their proliferation. Their sulfur compounds also support liver detoxification, which can benefit women dealing with hormonal imbalances linked to autoimmune conditions.

- Asparagus: Another excellent source of inulin, asparagus promotes digestive health and fosters a balanced microbiome by selectively feeding beneficial bacteria.

- Green Bananas: Containing resistant starch, green bananas act as a prebiotic by resisting digestion in the small intestine and reaching the colon, where they feed beneficial bacteria and encourage the production of SCFAs.

Combining Probiotics and Prebiotics: Synbiotic Foods Combining probiotics and prebiotics creates a "synbiotic" effect, where the prebiotic fibers feed the newly introduced probiotic bacteria, enhancing their survival and colonization in the gut. An example of a synbiotic food is a smoothie made with coconut yogurt (probiotic) and fibrous fruits like green bananas or apples (prebiotic). By consuming both probiotics and prebiotics together, women can optimize their gut health, support immune balance, and promote the production of anti-inflammatory compounds.

Supplementing with Prebiotics and Probiotics

In addition to dietary sources, women may consider taking probiotic and prebiotic supplements, particularly if dealing with digestive issues, chronic inflammation, or a history of antibiotic use that has disrupted the gut microbiome. Probiotic supplements with a variety of strains (multi-strain) and high colony-forming units (CFUs) can help re-establish a diverse microbiome. Prebiotic supplements, often containing inulin, fructooligosaccharides (FOS), or other soluble fibers, provide the necessary fuel for beneficial bacteria to thrive.

However, it's important to introduce these supplements gradually. Probiotics can initially cause mild digestive changes as the microbiome adjusts, and high doses of prebiotics may lead to gas and bloating if introduced too rapidly. Women should monitor their body's responses and adjust intake accordingly, potentially consulting with a healthcare provider to select strains or formulations tailored to their specific needs.

By thoughtfully incorporating both probiotics and prebiotics into their daily routine, women can support a resilient and balanced gut microbiome. This balance not only enhances digestive health but also plays a fundamental role in regulating the immune system, reducing inflammation, and promoting overall well-being in the context of autoimmune health.

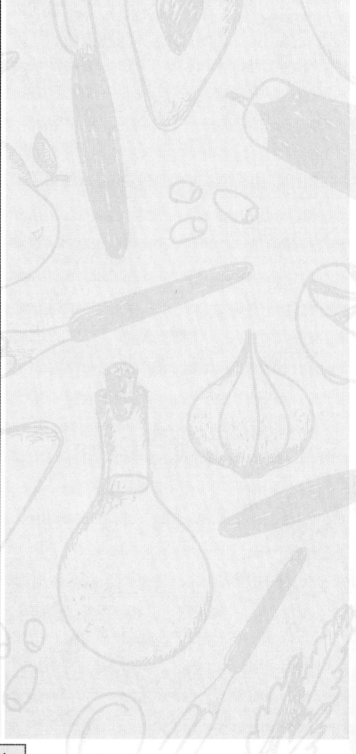

Chapter 8:
Pillar 4 – The Reintroduction Phase

The Reintroduction Phase is a critical step in the Autoimmune Protocol (AIP) diet, providing women with the opportunity to identify specific food triggers and tailor their diet for long-term health. After weeks of eliminating potentially inflammatory foods, the body has had time to reset, reduce inflammation, and heal the gut lining. This next phase is designed to systematically and carefully reintroduce foods that were initially removed, allowing for the detection of individual sensitivities. The reintroduction process not only fosters a deeper understanding of how different foods affect the body but also creates a more varied and sustainable diet over time. Utilizing a science-backed, structured approach, this phase enables women to pinpoint foods that support their health and those that may contribute to flare-ups. In this chapter, we delve into the strategies, timing, and careful monitoring required for a successful reintroduction, empowering women to build a personalized, balanced approach to their autoimmune wellness journey.

WHEN AND HOW TO REINTRODUCE FOODS

Reintroducing foods is a pivotal part of the AIP diet, allowing women to identify specific food sensitivities and expand their dietary options safely. The timing and method of reintroduction are crucial to ensure accurate results and to avoid inadvertently causing inflammation or autoimmune flare-ups. It's a systematic process that requires patience, careful observation, and a science-backed approach to truly understand how each food interacts with the body.

When to Begin the Reintroduction Phase

The Reintroduction Phase should commence only after a period of sustained symptom improvement during the Elimination Phase. Most women find that after 30 to 90 days of strictly following the AIP elimination guidelines, they experience a reduction in symptoms such as fatigue, joint pain, digestive issues, or skin flare-ups. This stabilization indicates that the gut has had sufficient time to heal and the immune system has calmed, creating an ideal baseline for reintroducing foods. Starting the reintroduction process prematurely, before experiencing any noticeable improvement, may cloud the identification of food triggers and compromise the integrity of the diet's healing benefits.

Women should also consider their lifestyle and stress levels before beginning the reintroduction. It is advisable to avoid reintroducing foods during periods of high stress, illness, or hormonal fluctuations, such as the menstrual cycle, as these factors can alter the body's response and make it difficult to accurately assess the effects of reintroduced foods. Choose a time when you can monitor your symptoms carefully and make the process a priority.

How to Reintroduce Foods: A Step-by-Step Guide

1. Select a Food to Reintroduce

Begin with foods that are less likely to trigger an immune response or cause inflammation. These typically include foods like egg yolks, certain nuts and seeds (like flaxseed or sunflower seeds), or high-quality dairy products such as ghee. Avoid starting with foods known to be common allergens or those with high inflammatory potential, like gluten or nightshade vegetables. The goal is to gradually reintroduce foods in an order that prioritizes those you may miss or find nutritionally beneficial, while minimizing the risk of triggering symptoms.

2. Start with a Small Amount

On the first day of reintroducing a food, consume a small amount, such as a teaspoon of the chosen item (e.g., a teaspoon of ghee or a small piece of nut). Wait 15 minutes and monitor for immediate reactions such as tingling in the mouth, digestive upset, or skin changes. If no adverse symptoms arise, proceed to the next step.

3. Gradually Increase the Amount

If there are no initial symptoms, consume a slightly larger portion of the food, such as a tablespoon or half a serving. Monitor your body's reaction for the next 2-3 hours. Look for delayed responses, which are common with food sensitivities. Symptoms to watch for include bloating, joint pain, fatigue, headaches, mood changes, or skin irritations. If no symptoms are observed, proceed to eat a regular-sized portion later in the day.

4. Wait 3 to 7 Days Before Introducing Another Food

Once you have reintroduced a food, avoid introducing any new foods for the next 3 to 7 days. This waiting period is crucial because food reactions can sometimes be delayed, and it may take a few days for symptoms to appear. During this period, continue to monitor your body's response. Keeping a detailed food journal can help track any changes in symptoms and provide insights into how your body is reacting to the newly reintroduced food.

5. Assess Your Response

If no adverse reactions occur during the waiting period, you can safely consider the food as well-tolerated and include it in your regular diet. However, if symptoms appear, this indicates a potential sensitivity, and the food should be avoided for a longer period before possibly reattempting reintroduction. Remember, the body's tolerance can change over time as the gut continues to heal, so foods that initially trigger symptoms may not always do so in the future.

6. <u>Repeat the Process with New Foods</u>

After completing the waiting period without any negative reactions, you can proceed to reintroduce the next food. Always start with the smallest possible amount and gradually increase, following the same systematic approach. It's essential to introduce only one food at a time to accurately determine its impact on your body.

Tips for a Successful Reintroduction

- <u>Use a Food Journal</u>: Document every reintroduction, noting the food, the quantity consumed, the time, and any symptoms experienced. This practice helps identify patterns and provides clarity on which foods are well-tolerated.

- <u>Introduce Whole, Unprocessed Foods</u>: During reintroduction, choose whole foods in their least processed forms to accurately gauge your body's response. Avoid processed versions of foods that may contain additives, preservatives, or hidden allergens, as these could confound your results.

- <u>Listen to Your Body</u>: The reintroduction process is highly individual. What works for one person may not work for another. Pay close attention to your body's signals, and do not rush the process.

The Science of Reintroduction

The methodical reintroduction of foods allows the immune system and gut to gradually encounter potential triggers in a controlled manner. By exposing the body to single foods at a time, you can assess its ability to tolerate them without overwhelming the immune system. This approach helps to identify foods that cause an overactive immune response, which could manifest as a flare-up of autoimmune symptoms. By avoiding these specific triggers, you create a personalized diet that supports long-term immune balance and well-being.

In summary, the reintroduction phase is about patience and precision. By adhering to a structured process, women can gain valuable insights into their unique food sensitivities and build a balanced, sustainable dietary plan that aligns with their health needs and lifestyle.

MONITORING AND TRACKING YOUR BODY'S RESPONSES

Monitoring your body's responses during the Reintroduction Phase is crucial for identifying specific food sensitivities and fine-tuning your diet for optimal health. For women with autoimmune conditions, subtle changes in symptoms can provide significant insights into how the body reacts to reintroduced foods. Tracking these responses not only empowers you to make informed dietary decisions but also contributes to long-term symptom management and overall well-being. This process relies on a careful blend of observation, documentation, and analysis, ensuring that the foods you incorporate into your diet support, rather than hinder, your health.

The Importance of Symptom Tracking

Autoimmune responses to food can manifest in various forms, ranging from digestive discomfort to joint pain, fatigue, skin issues, and mood changes. Some reactions may be immediate, occurring within minutes to a few hours, while others are delayed, emerging days after consumption. Due to this complexity, it is essential to monitor your body's signals systematically and over an extended period. By diligently tracking your symptoms, you can identify patterns that indicate intolerance or sensitivity to specific foods, allowing you to make more informed decisions about your dietary choices.

Research indicates that keeping a detailed symptom journal can significantly improve self-management of autoimmune conditions. In one study, individuals who consistently monitored their symptoms were more successful in identifying dietary triggers and experienced fewer flare-ups over time. For women, whose autoimmune symptoms can be influenced by factors such as hormonal fluctuations, tracking responses provides a clearer picture of how different foods interact with their unique physiological changes.

Creating a Symptom and Food Journal

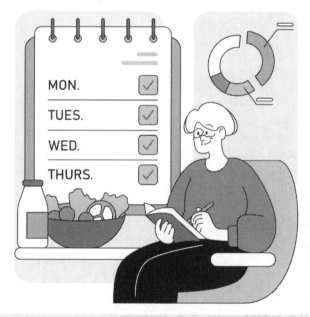

A symptom and food journal is an effective tool for capturing the nuances of your body's responses. Here's how to structure your journal for maximum insight:

1. Document Food Intake

Record each food you introduce, including the type of food, quantity, and time of consumption. Be specific— note the exact ingredients, preparation methods, and serving sizes. For example, instead of writing "nuts," specify "one tablespoon of almond butter." This level of detail will help you identify specific food components that might trigger a reaction.

2. Monitor Immediate and Delayed Responses

Divide your journal entries into short-term (0–3 hours) and long-term (1–3 days) observations. Immediate responses, such as digestive discomfort, skin reactions, or headaches, often indicate a more acute intolerance. Conversely, delayed responses, like joint pain, fatigue, mood changes, or changes in sleep patterns, may suggest a subtler, slower immune reaction. Tracking both types of responses is crucial for a comprehensive understanding of how your body interacts with reintroduced foods.

3. Use a Symptom Checklist

Create a checklist of common symptoms to monitor, focusing on those most relevant to your condition. Examples include:

- Digestive symptoms: bloating, gas, cramps, diarrhea, constipation.

- Skin changes: rashes, hives, acne, dryness.

- Joint and muscle pain: stiffness, swelling, aches.

- Neurological and mood-related symptoms: brain fog, anxiety, irritability, mood swings.

- Fatigue levels: changes in energy throughout the day, sleep quality.

Mark the presence and severity of each symptom on a scale (e.g., 0–5, where 0 is no symptoms and 5 is severe). This systematic approach allows you to quantify your reactions and track patterns over time.

4. Track Additional Influencing Factors

Include other factors that could affect your symptoms, such as stress levels, menstrual cycle phase, physical activity, sleep quality, and hydration. These factors can interact with your body's responses to food, providing a more comprehensive picture of how different elements impact your health. For example, you might notice that certain foods are better tolerated during the follicular phase of your cycle compared to the luteal phase, which could influence your reintroduction strategy.

Analyzing Your Data for Patterns

After reintroducing each food, review your journal entries to identify trends. Look for consistent symptom patterns linked to specific foods. For example, if you notice increased joint stiffness or skin rashes within 24– 48 hours of consuming a particular food, this may indicate a sensitivity. Similarly, if you experience digestive discomfort shortly after eating a new food, it might suggest an intolerance.

It is also helpful to compare symptom severity across different foods. If some foods cause a mild reaction while others result in more significant symptoms, you can prioritize which foods to avoid or limit in your long-term diet.

Using Technology for Tracking

Digital tools, such as food and symptom tracking apps, can facilitate this process by allowing you to log food intake and symptoms easily. Some apps even offer graphical data representations, making it simpler to identify patterns over time. Additionally, these tools can store a larger volume of data, enabling more detailed and long-term tracking that can provide valuable insights into your dietary responses.

Regular Check-Ins with a Healthcare Professional

Consider scheduling regular check-ins with a healthcare professional, such as a registered dietitian or a nutritionist specializing in autoimmune conditions. Sharing your food and symptom journal with a professional can provide an objective perspective and help interpret complex patterns. They can guide you in making informed decisions about reintroduction and help tailor your diet to support your unique health needs.

Adjusting Based on Your Findings

The primary goal of monitoring and tracking is to craft a personalized diet that aligns with your body's needs. If a food consistently causes adverse symptoms, it should remain off your regular menu. Conversely, foods that do not trigger symptoms can be incorporated into your diet, providing nutritional variety and balance. Remember that your body's responses may change over time, especially as gut healing progresses, so ongoing tracking remains beneficial even after the initial reintroduction phase.

By adopting a systematic, science-backed approach to monitoring your body's responses, you empower yourself to create a diet that not only minimizes symptoms but also promotes long-term health and well- being. This self-awareness becomes a powerful tool in managing autoimmune conditions, allowing women to take proactive steps toward a more balanced, symptom- free life.

Chapter 9:
Pillar 5 – Managing Stress Effectively

Managing stress is a critical pillar in the Autoimmune Protocol (AIP) diet, especially for women navigating the complexities of autoimmune conditions. Research has long established a connection between chronic stress and immune system dysregulation, revealing that prolonged stress can exacerbate inflammation, trigger symptom flare-ups, and hinder the healing process. For women, stress can have an even more pronounced impact due to the interplay between hormonal cycles and immune responses. Elevated cortisol levels, resulting from chronic stress, can disrupt the balance of the gut microbiome, compromise the intestinal barrier, and heighten autoimmunity. This chapter delves into evidence-based strategies for managing stress, highlighting practices such as mindfulness, yoga, deep breathing, and adequate sleep. By incorporating these techniques into daily life, women can create a more resilient immune system, reduce inflammation, and support the overall efficacy of the AIP diet in restoring health and well-being.

THE STRESS-AUTOIMMUNE CONNECTION

The link between stress and autoimmune conditions is well-documented, with research demonstrating that chronic stress can both trigger and exacerbate autoimmune responses. For women, this connection is particularly significant due to the intricate interplay between stress, hormonal fluctuations, and the immune system. Understanding the stress-autoimmune connection is crucial for effectively managing symptoms and supporting overall health.

When the body perceives stress—whether physical, emotional, or psychological—it activates the hypothalamic-pituitary-adrenal (HPA) axis. This triggers the release of cortisol, the body's primary stress hormone. In the short term, cortisol has anti-inflammatory effects and aids in modulating the immune response. However, chronic stress leads to consistently elevated cortisol levels, which can have the opposite effect, impairing immune regulation and promoting inflammation. Studies have shown that elevated cortisol disrupts the delicate balance between pro-inflammatory and anti-inflammatory cytokines, tipping the scale towards a heightened inflammatory state that is particularly problematic for individuals with autoimmune conditions.

One of the key ways stress impacts autoimmune conditions is through its effects on the gut microbiome and gut barrier integrity. Chronic stress has been found to alter the composition of gut bacteria, favoring the growth of pathogenic species while reducing beneficial bacteria. This state of dysbiosis compromises the gut's immune function, making it more vulnerable to inflammation. Additionally, stress increases the production of corticotropin-releasing hormone (CRH), which can enhance intestinal permeability, commonly known as "leaky gut." When the gut barrier is compromised, harmful substances like toxins, undigested food particles, and microbial fragments can leak into the bloodstream, triggering an immune response that may result in symptom flare-ups or the progression of autoimmunity.

For women, the stress-autoimmune connection is further complicated by the influence of hormonal fluctuations. Estrogen and progesterone, two primary female hormones, interact with the immune system in complex ways. During periods of high stress, the body's hormonal balance can shift, leading to changes in immune activity. For instance, high cortisol levels can interfere with estrogen metabolism, disrupting the body's natural hormonal cycles and potentially intensifying autoimmune symptoms. This is particularly relevant for women with conditions like Hashimoto's thyroiditis, rheumatoid arthritis, and lupus, where symptoms often worsen during times of stress or hormonal change, such as menstruation, pregnancy, or menopause.

Additionally, stress impacts the regulatory T-cells (Tregs), which play a critical role in maintaining immune tolerance by suppressing excessive immune responses. Chronic stress has been shown to reduce the number and function of Tregs, weakening the body's ability to control inappropriate immune attacks on its tissues. For women with autoimmune conditions, this can lead to an increase in symptom severity, including inflammation, joint pain, fatigue, and other debilitating effects.

Moreover, chronic stress can impair the body's ability to recover and heal. Elevated cortisol levels interfere with sleep quality, reducing the duration of deep, restorative sleep. Since deep sleep is essential for tissue repair, hormonal regulation, and the production of anti-inflammatory molecules, poor sleep further contributes to a cycle of immune dysfunction and inflammation.

In summary, the stress-autoimmune connection is a multifaceted relationship involving immune dysregulation, gut health, hormonal balance, and sleep quality. For women, managing stress effectively is not merely a matter of psychological well-being; it is a critical component of autoimmune health. By addressing stress through targeted interventions such as mindfulness practices, adequate sleep, and lifestyle adjustments, women can positively influence their immune response, reduce inflammation, and create a more conducive environment for healing and long-term disease management.

MINDFULNESS, MEDITATION, AND RELAXATION TECHNIQUES

Mindfulness, meditation, and relaxation techniques are scientifically supported methods for managing stress and promoting overall well-being, particularly for women dealing with autoimmune conditions. These practices are not just about achieving a sense of calm; they directly influence the body's physiological processes, including immune regulation, inflammation control, and hormonal balance. By integrating these techniques into daily life, women can mitigate the impact of chronic stress, reduce symptom flare-ups, and support the healing goals of the Autoimmune Protocol (AIP) diet.

The Science Behind Mindfulness and Meditation

Mindfulness involves focusing on the present moment with a non-judgmental attitude, allowing individuals to become aware of their thoughts, emotions, and physical sensations without being overwhelmed by them. Scientific research has shown that mindfulness practice can lead to changes in brain structure and function. Studies using neuroimaging techniques have found that regular mindfulness meditation increases the gray matter density in the prefrontal cortex, an area of the brain associated with emotional regulation, decision-making, and stress management.

The practice of mindfulness also engages the parasympathetic nervous system (PNS), which is responsible for the body's "rest and digest" responses. This activation counteracts the "fight or flight" response triggered by chronic stress and high cortisol levels, promoting a state of relaxation that supports immune function. For women with autoimmune conditions, a balanced immune system is crucial. Mindfulness meditation has been shown to reduce the production of pro-inflammatory cytokines, such as interleukin-6 (IL-6) and tumor necrosis factor-alpha (TNF-α), which are often elevated in autoimmune disorders. By lowering these inflammatory markers, meditation helps in alleviating symptoms such as joint pain, fatigue, and digestive issues.

Benefits of Mindfulness for Women with Autoimmunity

For women, who often juggle multiple roles and responsibilities, practicing mindfulness can bring a heightened awareness of the body's signals and needs. This awareness facilitates a better understanding of how stressors and emotional states affect autoimmune symptoms. Furthermore, by regularly engaging in

mindfulness, women can break the cycle of negative thought patterns and stress that may

CREATING A DAILY ROUTINE TO REDUCE STRESS

Establishing a structured daily routine is a powerful tool for managing stress, particularly for women with autoimmune conditions. A consistent routine helps regulate the body's internal clock, support hormonal balance, and promote healthy immune function. Stress reduction is vital in autoimmune health management, as it can reduce inflammatory responses, improve gut health, and enhance overall well-being. Incorporating specific science-backed practices into a daily schedule can create a framework that fosters resilience against stressors and minimizes symptom flare-ups.

Morning Rituals: Setting a Positive Tone for the Day

Starting the day with a calming morning routine sets a positive tone and reduces the likelihood of stress-induced cortisol spikes. Research suggests that engaging in a brief period of mindfulness meditation or deep breathing exercises upon waking can activate the parasympathetic nervous system, which lowers cortisol levels and prepares the body for a more balanced day. A 5-10 minute session focusing on slow, controlled breathing or a simple meditation practice can improve mood, enhance focus, and provide a sense of control that carries through the day.

Hydration is another critical morning habit. Drinking a glass of water shortly after waking helps rehydrate the body, supporting metabolic functions and cognitive clarity. Staying hydrated is linked to a reduction in stress-related symptoms, such as headaches and fatigue, which can be particularly bothersome for women managing autoimmune conditions.

Incorporating gentle movement in the morning, such as stretching, yoga, or a short walk, can boost circulation, alleviate joint stiffness, and release endorphins—natural chemicals in the brain that act as stress relievers. Studies show that low-impact exercise can enhance mood and reduce markers of inflammation, making it a beneficial routine for women with autoimmune disorders.

Structured Meals and Breaks: Supporting Gut and Hormonal Health

The timing and composition of meals play a significant role in stress management. Establishing regular meal times helps regulate blood sugar levels, preventing dips that can trigger stress responses and inflammation. Women with autoimmune conditions should aim for nutrient-dense, balanced meals that include healthy fats, high-quality protein, and fiber-rich vegetables. This combination supports steady energy release, hormone regulation, and gut health.

Integrating mindful eating into each meal encourages a focus on the present moment, reducing stress-induced digestive issues. Taking time to savor food, chewing slowly, and appreciating the sensory aspects of the meal can improve digestion and nutrient absorption, which are often compromised in individuals with autoimmune conditions. A mindful eating practice has been linked to reductions in cortisol levels and improvements in digestive health.

Scheduling short breaks throughout the day, especially during work or caregiving responsibilities, is essential for stress management. These breaks provide an opportunity to reset the mind and body. Research indicates that incorporating brief periods of relaxation, such as stretching, deep breathing, or listening to calming music, can lower heart rate, decrease muscle tension, and reduce mental fatigue. For women with autoimmune conditions, these mini-breaks can prevent the accumulation of stress, which can otherwise lead to symptom exacerbation.

Evening Wind-Down Routine: Preparing for Restorative Sleep

An evening routine designed to wind down the body and mind is crucial for promoting quality sleep, a key component in managing autoimmune health. The blue light emitted by screens from phones, computers, and televisions interferes with melatonin production, a hormone that regulates sleep-wake cycles. Limiting screen time at least an hour before bed and opting for activities such as reading a book, listening to calming music, or practicing relaxation techniques can prepare the body for restful sleep.

Epsom salt baths are a soothing addition to an evening routine. Epsom salts contain magnesium sulfate, which can be absorbed through the skin and may help relax muscles and improve sleep quality. Magnesium also plays a role in regulating the nervous system, aiding in the reduction of anxiety and stress. Studies have shown that regular magnesium supplementation can improve sleep, reduce muscle pain, and alleviate fatigue, which are common issues for women with autoimmune conditions.

Journaling is another effective wind-down practice. Taking a few minutes each evening to write down thoughts, feelings, and experiences helps process the events of the day, reduce mental clutter, and identify stressors. Research suggests that expressive writing can improve mental health by lowering cortisol levels and enhancing emotional regulation. Women with autoimmune conditions can use this practice to track symptoms, identify triggers, and reflect on their stress management strategies.

Consistency and Adaptation: Keys to Routine Success

Consistency is the cornerstone of an effective stress-reducing routine. The body thrives on regularity, as predictable patterns help regulate circadian rhythms, hormone release, and digestive processes. However, it is also essential to remain flexible and adapt the routine to suit changing circumstances. For instance, during times of increased stress or hormonal shifts, such as menstrual cycles, women may benefit from adjusting the intensity of physical activities or incorporating additional relaxation practices.

Over time, a structured daily routine that integrates mindful practices, balanced nutrition, hydration, gentle movement, and intentional relaxation can build resilience against stress, supporting immune regulation and promoting overall well-being. This holistic approach not only reduces daily stress but also lays the foundation for long-term management of autoimmune conditions, allowing women to feel more in control of their health.

Chapter 10:
Pillar 6 – Prioritizing Sleep and Recovery

Sleep and recovery are often overlooked yet vital components in the management of autoimmune conditions, particularly for women. Research shows that sleep is intricately linked with immune function, hormonal balance, and gut health. During deep sleep, the body enters a state of repair, producing anti-inflammatory molecules and regulating stress hormones such as cortisol. For women managing autoimmune disorders, prioritizing sleep can have a profound impact on symptom relief, mental clarity, and overall well-being. This chapter delves into the science of sleep, highlighting its role in reducing inflammation, supporting a balanced immune response, and promoting optimal gut health. We will explore evidence-based strategies to improve sleep quality, address common sleep disturbances associated with autoimmunity, and establish routines that encourage restorative rest. By prioritizing sleep and recovery, women can enhance the efficacy of the Autoimmune Protocol (AIP) diet and build a solid foundation for long-term healing and resilience.

SLEEP'S CRITICAL ROLE IN IMMUNE FUNCTION

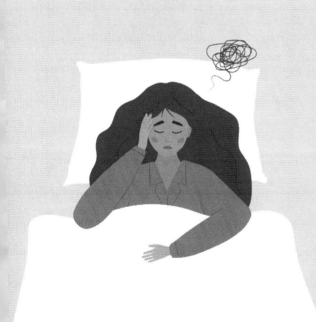

Sleep plays a pivotal role in maintaining a well-regulated immune system, which is particularly important for women with autoimmune conditions. The relationship between sleep and immunity is bidirectional: while the immune system influences sleep patterns, sleep also affects how efficiently the immune system functions. Understanding this interplay is essential for managing autoimmune symptoms and promoting overall health.

During sleep, especially in the deep stages (slow-wave sleep), the body undergoes a variety of processes that are crucial for immune regulation. One key process is the production and release of cytokines, small proteins that act as signaling molecules in the immune system. Certain cytokines, such as interleukin-6 (IL-6) and tumor necrosis factor-alpha (TNF-α), are known to increase in response to infections or inflammation. Sleep helps regulate the balance of pro-inflammatory and anti-inflammatory cytokines, ensuring that the body can effectively respond to potential threats without tipping into a state of chronic inflammation. For women with autoimmune conditions, achieving this balance is critical, as excessive production of pro-inflammatory cytokines can exacerbate symptoms and lead to flare-ups.

Another important immune-related function of sleep is the enhancement of T-cell activity. T-cells are a type of white blood cell that play a central role in the body's adaptive immune response. They help identify and destroy pathogens, infected cells, and other foreign invaders. Research has shown that during sleep, the body increases T-cell production and function, facilitating a more effective immune response. In contrast, chronic sleep deprivation has been linked to a reduction in T-cell activity, potentially weakening the body's ability to regulate immune responses. This weakened regulation can contribute to the overactive immune responses characteristic of autoimmune diseases, such as rheumatoid arthritis, lupus, and Hashimoto's thyroiditis.

Sleep is also essential for the regulation of the hypothalamic-pituitary-adrenal (HPA) axis, which controls the body's stress response through the release of cortisol. Adequate sleep helps modulate cortisol levels, keeping them within a healthy range. Since cortisol has immunomodulatory effects, helping to suppress excessive immune activity, a well-regulated sleep-wake cycle supports a balanced immune function. However, poor sleep disrupts this balance, leading to elevated cortisol levels, which can further contribute to immune dysregulation and inflammation. For women, who may experience hormonal fluctuations that already affect cortisol levels, maintaining good sleep hygiene becomes even more crucial to support immune health and reduce the risk of autoimmune flare-ups.

Furthermore, sleep supports the maintenance of the gut barrier and the microbiome, both of which are closely linked to immune function. Research indicates that sleep deprivation can alter the gut microbiome, promoting dysbiosis, which can compromise gut barrier integrity and lead to increased intestinal permeability (commonly known as "leaky gut"). This leaky gut allows toxins and undigested food particles to enter the bloodstream, triggering immune responses that can exacerbate autoimmune symptoms. Therefore, by prioritizing quality sleep, women can promote gut health, which in turn positively impacts the immune system.

The natural sleep-wake cycle, also known as the circadian rhythm, further plays a role in synchronizing various immune functions. The production of certain immune cells, including natural killer (NK) cells, peaks at specific times of the day in alignment with the body's circadian clock. Disruptions to this rhythm—whether due to irregular sleep patterns, shift work, or stress—can interfere with the optimal timing of immune responses, leading to heightened inflammation and impaired ability to fend off pathogens. Women with autoimmune conditions often have more sensitive immune systems, and thus maintaining a regular sleep schedule is key to supporting the body's natural immune rhythm.

In summary, sleep is far more than a period of physical rest; it is an active process that supports the body's immune regulation, reduces inflammation, and promotes gut health. For women managing autoimmune conditions, prioritizing sleep not only helps reduce symptom severity but also builds a foundation for improved immune balance. By understanding and addressing the critical role of sleep in immune function, women can take meaningful steps toward enhancing their health and resilience.

TIPS FOR IMPROVING SLEEP QUALITY

Quality sleep is essential for regulating the immune system, managing inflammation, and supporting overall well-being, particularly for women with autoimmune conditions. However, many factors—such as stress, hormonal fluctuations, and inflammation—can disrupt sleep patterns. Implementing science-backed strategies to improve sleep quality can significantly impact symptom management and enhance the body's natural healing processes. Here are several evidence-based tips to help improve sleep quality and create a sleep-conducive environment.

1. Maintain a Consistent Sleep Schedule

Sticking to a regular sleep-wake schedule, even on weekends, helps regulate the body's circadian rhythm—the internal clock that governs the sleep-wake cycle. A consistent routine reinforces the body's natural rhythm, facilitating the release of sleep-promoting hormones like melatonin. Research indicates that irregular sleep patterns can lead to disruptions in circadian rhythms, which not only affect sleep quality but also impair immune function and increase inflammation. For women, establishing a routine that aligns with their natural circadian rhythm can support hormonal balance, reduce autoimmune flare-ups, and improve overall health.

2. Create a Sleep-Inducing Environment

The sleep environment plays a crucial role in promoting deep, restorative sleep. To enhance sleep quality, ensure that the bedroom is cool, dark, and quiet. The optimal room temperature for sleep is between 60-67°F (15-19°C), as cooler temperatures facilitate the body's natural drop in core temperature, signaling it is time to sleep. Using blackout curtains or an eye mask can help block out light, which interferes with melatonin production, while earplugs or white noise machines can minimize noise disturbances.

Investing in a comfortable mattress and pillows suited to your sleeping position can also make a significant difference. Studies show that poor mattress quality can lead to discomfort and disrupted sleep, which can be particularly challenging for women with joint pain or fibromyalgia associated with autoimmune conditions.

3. Limit Exposure to Blue Light in the Evening

Exposure to blue light from electronic devices such as phones, computers, and televisions in the evening can suppress melatonin production, making it more difficult to fall asleep. To mitigate this effect, avoid screens at least 1-2 hours before bedtime. Instead, consider engaging in relaxing activities like reading, listening to calming music, or practicing mindfulness exercises. If avoiding screens is not possible, consider using blue-light-blocking glasses or enabling the "night mode" setting on devices to reduce blue light exposure.

4. Develop a Relaxing Pre-Sleep Routine

Creating a relaxing pre-sleep routine helps signal to the body that it is time to wind down. Incorporating deep breathing exercises, meditation, or gentle yoga into this routine can activate the parasympathetic nervous system, lowering cortisol levels and preparing the body for rest. A warm bath with Epsom salts can also be beneficial; the magnesium in Epsom salts is absorbed through the skin and has been shown to promote muscle relaxation and alleviate tension, easing the transition into sleep.

For women, particularly those experiencing hormonal fluctuations that may interfere with sleep, integrating aromatherapy into the pre-sleep routine can be helpful. Essential oils like lavender and chamomile have been shown to have sedative effects, reducing anxiety and improving sleep quality. Adding a few drops to a diffuser or using a pillow spray can enhance relaxation.

5. Be Mindful of Diet and Hydration

What you consume throughout the day can significantly affect sleep quality. Avoid caffeine and nicotine at least 4-6 hours before bedtime, as both are stimulants that can interfere with the ability to fall asleep and achieve deep sleep. Similarly, large meals and spicy foods close to bedtime can cause discomfort or indigestion, disrupting sleep. If hunger strikes in the evening, opt for a light snack that includes sleep-supportive nutrients, such as a small handful of nuts or a banana, both of which contain magnesium and tryptophan to aid in relaxation.

Hydration is essential, but it's advisable to limit fluid intake in the hour or two before bed to reduce nighttime awakenings caused by the need to use the restroom.

6. Get Exposure to Natural Light During the Day

Daytime exposure to natural sunlight helps regulate the circadian rhythm by signaling to the body when it is time to be awake. Aim to spend time outside during the morning hours, even if it's just for a short walk. Natural light boosts serotonin production, which not only enhances mood but also converts to melatonin in the evening, aiding in sleep. This practice is particularly helpful for women with autoimmune conditions who may experience disruptions in their sleep-wake cycle due to hormonal imbalances or chronic inflammation.

7. Incorporate Supplements Wisely

Certain natural supplements can support sleep quality, but they should be used thoughtfully and ideally under the guidance of a healthcare professional. Magnesium is known for its calming effects on the nervous system and can aid in sleep for women experiencing muscle cramps or stress. Melatonin supplements can be helpful, especially for those who have difficulty falling asleep due to a disrupted sleep-wake cycle. However, it's important to use melatonin sparingly, as long-term or high-dose use can potentially disrupt the body's natural hormone production.

Herbal supplements like valerian root, chamomile, and passionflower have also been found to support sleep by reducing anxiety and promoting relaxation. While generally considered safe, these supplements should be used with caution and tailored to individual needs, especially when managing autoimmune conditions.

8. Practice Stress-Reduction Techniques Throughout the Day

Daytime stress management has a direct impact on sleep quality. Incorporating mindfulness practices, regular physical activity, and relaxation techniques into your daily routine helps to keep stress levels in check, making it easier to unwind at night. For women dealing with autoimmune conditions, finding stress-relief strategies that work, such as spending time in nature, practicing gratitude, or engaging in creative activities, can enhance both mental well-being and sleep quality.

By implementing these evidence-based strategies, women can significantly improve their sleep quality, providing the body with the rest it needs to support immune regulation, hormonal balance, and overall health. Prioritizing sleep as part of an integrated approach to the Autoimmune Protocol (AIP) diet can help women feel more energized, reduce symptom severity, and contribute to long-term healing.

UNDERSTANDING YOUR BODY'S SIGNALS FOR REST

Understanding your body's signals for rest is an essential skill, particularly for women managing autoimmune conditions. Your body communicates when it needs downtime to repair and restore itself, and learning to interpret these signals can significantly impact your health and symptom management. Autoimmune diseases often push the body into a constant state of overactivity, which can make recognizing the need for rest more challenging. However, ignoring these signals can lead to exacerbated symptoms, prolonged inflammation, and delayed healing. Therefore, it is crucial to become attuned to these cues and respond appropriately to promote a balanced immune system and overall well-being.

Recognizing Physical Fatigue

One of the primary signals the body uses to indicate a need for rest is physical fatigue. This type of fatigue is not just the tiredness that follows a long day; it is a deep sense of exhaustion that affects the muscles, joints, and even cognitive function. In women with autoimmune conditions, physical fatigue often accompanies activities that previously would not have been strenuous. This can include simple daily tasks like grocery shopping, light exercise, or even social interactions.

Research shows that physical fatigue in autoimmune diseases, such as lupus or rheumatoid arthritis, is linked to the body's chronic inflammatory state. Cytokines released during inflammation can affect muscle function, disrupt energy metabolism, and impact the nervous system, leading to a profound sense of tiredness. If you notice that regular activities are increasingly draining or that it takes longer to recover from physical exertion, your body is signaling the need for more rest and a lighter activity load.

Listening to Cognitive Signs: Brain Fog and Mental Fatigue

Brain fog is a common and often overlooked signal that the body needs rest. This condition is characterized by a sense of mental cloudiness, difficulty concentrating, memory lapses, and slower cognitive processing. Autoimmune conditions frequently disrupt normal cognitive functions due to ongoing inflammation, changes in hormone levels, and alterations in neurotransmitter activity.

Women are particularly susceptible to experiencing brain fog during periods of hormonal fluctuation, such as menstruation or menopause, which can further exacerbate autoimmune symptoms. Studies have shown that chronic inflammation in the body can affect the central nervous system and brain function, leading to cognitive impairments. If you find yourself struggling to focus, forgetting routine tasks, or feeling mentally sluggish, it is your body's way of signaling a need for a mental break or more sleep. Engaging in a brief rest period, mindfulness exercises, or a quiet, low-stimulation activity can help alleviate cognitive fatigue.

Emotional and Mood Cues

Emotional fluctuations, such as irritability, heightened anxiety, or sudden mood swings, are also key indicators that the body is under stress and requires rest. When the body is fatigued or overwhelmed by chronic inflammation, it can affect the hypothalamic-pituitary-adrenal (HPA) axis, which regulates the stress response and cortisol production. Elevated cortisol levels, resulting from prolonged stress, can negatively impact mood and emotional stability, leaving you feeling on edge or more susceptible to anxiety and emotional outbursts.

Women often juggle multiple roles and responsibilities, which can further compound emotional stress, particularly when managing an autoimmune condition. When feelings of irritability or emotional exhaustion surface, it is a sign that the body is signaling for a pause. Incorporating relaxation techniques such as deep breathing, yoga, or simply allowing yourself a quiet moment can help reset your emotional state and prevent further stress-induced inflammation.

Sleep Disruptions: A Signal of Imbalance

Sleep disturbances, including difficulty falling asleep, staying asleep, or experiencing non-restorative sleep, can be both a cause and a symptom of an underlying imbalance in the body's need for rest. When sleep quality is compromised, the body's natural repair processes, hormone regulation, and immune modulation are disrupted, often resulting in increased fatigue during the day.

For women, these sleep disruptions can sometimes be linked to hormonal changes, such as fluctuating levels of estrogen and progesterone, which influence sleep patterns and circadian rhythm. Additionally, autoimmune conditions can lead to increased pain or discomfort at night, further affecting the ability to rest adequately. If you find yourself waking up tired or struggling with sleep consistency, this is an indicator that your body is not getting the restorative rest it requires. Addressing sleep hygiene, such as setting a consistent sleep schedule, limiting screen time before bed, and creating a calming nighttime routine, can help mitigate these disturbances.

Digestive Discomfort as a Rest Cue

Digestive symptoms, such as bloating, indigestion, or changes in bowel movements, can be another subtle signal that the body needs to slow down. Stress and lack of rest can negatively impact gut motility and the gut-brain axis, leading to disrupted digestion and altered gut microbiome composition. When the body is overwhelmed, it may divert energy away from digestion to prioritize other systems, resulting in digestive discomfort.

In women, this can be further influenced by hormonal changes that affect gut motility and enzyme activity. If you notice that digestive discomfort worsens during periods of physical or emotional strain, it may be time to heed these signs and incorporate more rest into your daily routine. Gentle activities like mindful eating, relaxation exercises, and consuming gut-supportive foods can help ease digestive symptoms and restore balance.

Responding to Your Body's Signals

Learning to listen to these physical, cognitive, and emotional signals is essential in managing autoimmune conditions. When you become attuned to these cues, you can take proactive steps to adjust your activity levels, incorporate rest periods, and practice self-care techniques that promote recovery. Importantly, responding to your body's need for rest does not mean inactivity; it means finding the balance between activity and recuperation that suits your unique needs.

Incorporating regular check-ins throughout the day, where you pause to assess how you feel physically and mentally, can help you become more in sync with your body's needs. By acknowledging these signals and making rest a priority, you create an environment that supports immune regulation, reduces inflammation, and fosters a path toward greater health and vitality.

Chapter 11:
Pillar 7 – Incorporating Physical Activity

Physical activity is a crucial yet nuanced pillar in the management of autoimmune conditions. While exercise is widely recognized for its benefits, including reducing inflammation, improving mood, and enhancing overall physical health, it must be approached thoughtfully by women with autoimmune diseases. Overexertion can trigger symptom flare-ups, while too little movement can lead to muscle stiffness, increased fatigue, and reduced mobility. Scientific research shows that moderate, consistent exercise can help regulate the immune system, support cardiovascular health, and improve mental well-being. This chapter explores how to incorporate physical activity into your routine in a way that respects the body's needs and promotes healing. We will discuss types of exercises best suited for women with autoimmune conditions, how to listen to your body's signals, and the importance of balancing activity with adequate rest. By integrating tailored physical activity, you can build strength, enhance flexibility, and support your journey toward optimal health.

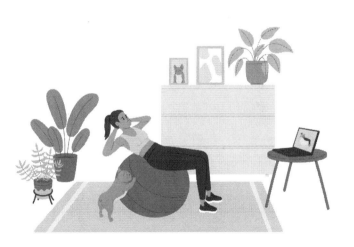

BENEFITS OF EXERCISE ON IMMUNE HEALTH

Exercise plays a fundamental role in maintaining a balanced and effective immune system, offering numerous benefits for women managing autoimmune conditions. While physical activity is known to support cardiovascular health and mental well-being, research has increasingly highlighted its positive impact on immune regulation. Regular, moderate exercise can reduce inflammation, enhance the body's ability to fight infections, and improve overall immune function. Understanding these benefits helps underscore the importance of integrating movement into a comprehensive autoimmune management plan.

1. Regulation of Inflammatory Responses

One of the key benefits of regular exercise is its ability to modulate the body's inflammatory responses. During and immediately after exercise, the body releases anti-inflammatory cytokines such as interleukin-10 (IL-10) and myokines, which are signaling proteins produced by muscle contractions. These molecules help to dampen chronic inflammation, which is particularly relevant for women with autoimmune diseases, where inflammation often drives symptom severity. Studies have shown that engaging in moderate-intensity activities, like walking, swimming, or yoga, can reduce levels of pro-inflammatory markers like interleukin-6 (IL-6) and C-reactive protein (CRP), aiding in symptom management and potentially reducing flare-ups.

2. Enhancement of Immune Surveillance

Exercise also boosts immune surveillance, the body's ability to detect and respond to pathogens and abnormal cells. Physical activity increases the circulation of white blood cells, particularly natural killer (NK) cells and T-cells, which play a critical role in immune defense. By promoting a higher turnover of these cells in the bloodstream, exercise enhances the body's capacity to identify and neutralize potential threats. For women with autoimmune conditions, an improved immune surveillance system can contribute to better overall immune balance, supporting the body's ability to defend against infections and regulate abnormal immune activity.

3. Support of Lymphatic Function

The lymphatic system is a crucial component of the immune system, responsible for transporting immune cells throughout the body and removing waste products, toxins, and pathogens. Unlike the cardiovascular system, the lymphatic system does not have a pump like the heart to facilitate circulation. Instead, muscle contractions during physical activity act as a pump for the lymphatic vessels, promoting the efficient movement of lymph fluid. By stimulating lymphatic circulation, exercise supports detoxification, enhances immune cell trafficking, and helps clear out inflammatory substances. This is particularly important for women managing conditions like rheumatoid arthritis or lupus, where lymphatic congestion can contribute to swelling and discomfort.

4. Improved Gut Health and the Gut-Immune Axis

Emerging research has demonstrated a strong link between physical activity and gut health, a critical aspect of immune function. Moderate exercise has been found to promote a more diverse gut microbiome, enhancing the population of beneficial bacteria that play a role in regulating the immune system and reducing intestinal permeability. A healthier gut microbiome can produce anti-inflammatory compounds, such as short-chain fatty acids (SCFAs), which strengthen the gut barrier and prevent unwanted substances from entering the bloodstream and triggering an immune response.

For women with autoimmune conditions like inflammatory bowel disease (IBD) or celiac disease, where gut health is directly linked to immune regulation, incorporating moderate exercise can help support the gut-immune axis. Improved gut health contributes to a more balanced immune response, reducing the risk of inflammation and autoimmunity flare-ups.

5. Hormonal Regulation and Stress Reduction

Exercise plays a significant role in regulating hormones, including cortisol, the body's primary stress hormone. Chronic stress can elevate cortisol levels, leading to immune dysregulation and increased inflammation. Regular physical activity has been shown to modulate cortisol production, reducing stress and promoting a state of relaxation. Activities such as yoga, tai chi, and light aerobic exercise not only enhance physical health but also support mental well-being by releasing endorphins—chemicals in the brain that act as natural painkillers and mood elevators.

For women, who often experience additional hormonal fluctuations due to menstrual cycles, pregnancy, and menopause, exercise can help stabilize hormone levels and support a more balanced immune response. This is especially beneficial for conditions like Hashimoto's thyroiditis and lupus, where hormone-immune interactions play a significant role in disease activity.

6. Enhanced Sleep Quality and Recovery

Another indirect benefit of regular exercise is the improvement of sleep quality, which is essential for immune health and recovery. Physical activity helps regulate the sleep-wake cycle, promoting deeper and more restorative sleep. Quality sleep is vital for the immune system, as it facilitates the production of cytokines that regulate immune responses and supports the repair and regeneration of tissues. Women managing autoimmune diseases often struggle with sleep disturbances, and incorporating exercise can help alleviate these issues, creating a positive feedback loop where improved sleep further enhances immune function.

7. Muscle Strength and Joint Health

For women with autoimmune conditions that affect the joints and muscles, such as rheumatoid arthritis and fibromyalgia, exercise improves muscle strength and joint flexibility. Stronger muscles provide better support to the joints, reducing strain and the risk of injury. Additionally, movement increases the production of synovial fluid, which lubricates the joints and enhances mobility, helping to alleviate stiffness and discomfort. By maintaining joint health, exercise enables women to stay active and avoid the cycle of inactivity and muscle deconditioning, which can exacerbate symptoms and impair immune regulation.

Finding the Right Balance

While exercise offers numerous benefits for immune health, it is important to strike a balance. High-intensity or excessive exercise can place stress on the body, potentially increasing inflammation and leading to symptom flare-ups in women with autoimmune conditions. The key is to engage in moderate-intensity activities tailored to your body's current capabilities and to incorporate rest periods to allow for recovery. Activities like walking, swimming, stretching, and low-impact strength training can provide the benefits of exercise without overtaxing the immune system.

By understanding the science-backed benefits of exercise on immune health and carefully incorporating it into a daily routine, women can enhance their body's natural defenses, reduce inflammation, and improve their quality of life.

CHOOSING THE RIGHT TYPE AND INTENSITY OF ACTIVITY

Selecting the appropriate type and intensity of physical activity is crucial for women managing autoimmune conditions. While exercise offers numerous benefits for immune health, choosing the wrong type or intensity can lead to overexertion, heightened inflammation, or even flare-ups. A tailored approach that considers individual health status, symptom severity, and energy levels is essential to maximize the benefits of exercise without compromising well-being. Scientific research has consistently shown that moderate-intensity activities are the most effective in promoting immune function, reducing inflammation, and supporting overall health in individuals with autoimmune disorders.

1. Starting with Low-Impact Activities

For women experiencing significant fatigue, joint pain, or muscle stiffness, starting with low-impact exercises is a safe and effective way to introduce physical activity. Low-impact activities, such as walking, swimming, cycling, yoga, and tai chi, are gentle on the joints and muscles while still providing the benefits of improved circulation, flexibility, and mood enhancement. These forms of exercise help activate the body's natural anti-inflammatory responses without placing excessive strain on the immune system.

- Walking: A simple yet effective activity, walking can be easily adjusted in intensity by varying the pace and distance. Research indicates that regular, brisk walking can reduce systemic inflammation and improve cardiovascular health. For those new to exercise, starting with short, 10-15 minute walks and gradually increasing duration as stamina improves can provide significant health benefits without causing undue stress.

- Swimming and Aquatic Therapy: Swimming and water-based exercises are especially beneficial for women with autoimmune conditions that affect the joints, such as rheumatoid arthritis or lupus. The buoyancy of water reduces the impact on joints, allowing for full-body movement and muscle strengthening with minimal pain. Additionally, water resistance provides a natural, low-intensity strength workout that supports muscle tone and joint flexibility.

- Yoga and Tai Chi: Both yoga and tai chi are mind-body practices that combine physical movement with breathing techniques and mindfulness. These exercises not only promote flexibility and balance but also help reduce stress and improve mental well-being. Scientific studies have found that yoga and tai chi can lower levels of cortisol, the stress hormone, and reduce markers of systemic inflammation. Women experiencing autoimmune symptoms such as joint stiffness, fatigue, and anxiety may find these practices particularly helpful in managing their condition.

2. Incorporating Strength Training

Once the body has adapted to low-impact activities, strength training can be gradually introduced to build muscle mass, support joint health, and enhance overall physical function. For women with autoimmune conditions, maintaining muscle strength is vital, as muscle weakness and wasting are common complications of chronic inflammation and inactivity. However, it is essential to approach strength training with caution, starting with light weights or resistance bands and focusing on proper form to prevent injury.

- Bodyweight Exercises: Simple bodyweight exercises, such as squats, lunges, push-ups, and planks, are excellent starting points. These exercises engage multiple muscle groups and can be modified to suit individual fitness levels. For example, performing push-ups against a wall or using a chair for support during squats can reduce the intensity while still providing muscle-strengthening benefits.

- Resistance Bands: Resistance bands offer a low-impact way to incorporate strength training without the need for heavy equipment. They provide controlled resistance throughout the range of motion,

helping to improve muscle strength and endurance. Studies suggest that resistance training using bands can enhance muscle tone and joint stability, which is especially beneficial for women with autoimmune conditions that affect mobility.

3. Monitoring Intensity Using the "Talk Test"

Choosing the right intensity is key to preventing overexertion, which can trigger fatigue, muscle soreness, and immune system dysregulation. One practical way to gauge exercise intensity is the "talk test": During moderate-intensity exercise, you should be able to carry on a conversation but may need to pause to take a breath. If you are unable to speak in full sentences, the exercise may be too intense. Conversely, if you can sing comfortably without needing to pause for breath, you may need to increase the intensity slightly to reach the moderate level.

For women with autoimmune conditions, the goal is to maintain a moderate-intensity level, which is associated with enhanced immune function and reduced inflammation. High-intensity activities, such as intense cardio or heavy weightlifting, may provoke a temporary suppression of the immune system, potentially leading to increased susceptibility to infections or symptom flare-ups. Therefore, it is generally advisable to focus on steady, moderate-intensity exercises that provide health benefits while allowing the body ample time to recover.

4. Building in Rest Days and Recovery Time

Incorporating regular rest days is essential for allowing the body to recover and repair itself, particularly for women managing autoimmune conditions. Overtraining can lead to immune suppression, muscle damage, and elevated levels of inflammatory markers, negating the benefits of exercise. A balanced routine typically includes 3-4 days of moderate exercise interspersed with rest days or days dedicated to light, restorative activities such as stretching, gentle yoga, or walking.

Listening to your body is crucial: If you experience increased fatigue, joint pain, or muscle soreness, it may be a sign to reduce intensity, shorten the duration of workouts, or take additional rest days. By respecting these signals, you create a sustainable exercise routine that supports, rather than hinders, your healing process.

5. Adjusting for Flare-Ups

Autoimmune conditions often involve periods of symptom flare-ups, during which exercise routines may need to be modified. During a flare-up, focus on gentle movement and relaxation techniques, such as deep breathing, meditation, or stretching. This approach helps maintain circulation and flexibility without placing additional stress on the body. Once symptoms subside, you can gradually resume your regular activity level, adjusting intensity based on how your body responds.

5. Consulting with a Healthcare Professional

Before starting any new exercise regimen, it is advisable to consult with a healthcare professional, particularly if you have specific limitations due to an autoimmune condition. A physical therapist or certified fitness trainer with experience in autoimmune health can provide tailored guidance, ensuring that your exercise plan aligns with your body's unique needs and capabilities.

In summary, the key to incorporating physical activity for women with autoimmune conditions is to choose the right type and intensity that promotes health without overtaxing the body. By selecting low-impact exercises, incorporating strength training thoughtfully, and respecting the body's signals, you can build a balanced routine that supports immune regulation, reduces inflammation, and enhances overall well-being.

MIND-BODY EXERCISES: YOGA, TAI CHI, AND MORE

Mind-body exercises like yoga, tai chi, and qigong have been widely recognized for their unique ability to address both the physical and mental aspects of health, making them especially beneficial for women managing autoimmune conditions. These practices combine gentle physical movements with controlled breathing, meditation, and mindfulness, offering a holistic approach to reducing stress, enhancing flexibility, and promoting immune balance. Research supports their role in alleviating inflammation, improving mood, and optimizing the body's self-healing mechanisms.

1. Yoga: Cultivating Strength and Calm

Yoga is an ancient practice that integrates physical postures, breath control, and meditation. It has gained popularity as a therapeutic exercise for managing chronic conditions, including autoimmune diseases. Yoga's emphasis on gentle stretching, balance, and controlled movements can be particularly beneficial for women experiencing joint pain, muscle stiffness, or fatigue.

Scientific studies have shown that regular yoga practice can lower cortisol levels and reduce pro-inflammatory cytokines, both of which are crucial in managing autoimmune conditions. The practice encourages the activation of the parasympathetic nervous system (the "rest and digest" state), helping to counterbalance the effects of chronic stress on the body. By enhancing relaxation, yoga can lead to a decrease in systemic inflammation, which may alleviate symptoms such as joint pain, brain fog, and fatigue.

- Gentle Forms of Yoga: For women with autoimmune conditions, choosing the right type of yoga is essential. Hatha yoga, yin yoga, and restorative yoga are gentle forms that focus on slow, deliberate movements and extended postures, promoting relaxation and flexibility without overexerting the body. These styles of yoga allow for modifications to suit individual comfort levels, making them accessible regardless of physical limitations.

- Breathwork and Meditation: Yoga places significant emphasis on pranayama (breathwork) and meditation, which play a key role in regulating the body's stress response. Deep, controlled breathing techniques enhance oxygenation, calm the nervous system, and reduce the production of stress hormones. Additionally, incorporating meditation into yoga practice fosters mental clarity, emotional regulation, and mindfulness, which can improve one's ability to cope with the challenges of autoimmune conditions.

2. Tai Chi: Enhancing Balance and Energy Flow

Tai chi, a form of martial art originating from ancient China, is characterized by slow, flowing movements that focus on balance, body awareness, and mental tranquility. Often referred to as "meditation in motion," tai chi integrates physical exercise with mindfulness, making it a suitable activity for women seeking to improve physical health and manage stress without excessive physical strain.

Clinical research has highlighted tai chi's impact on immune modulation and inflammation control. In a study involving patients with rheumatoid arthritis, tai chi practice was found to significantly reduce levels of inflammatory markers and improve joint mobility. The gentle, rhythmic movements of tai chi stimulate the lymphatic system, enhancing circulation and supporting the body's natural detoxification processes. This is especially beneficial for women with autoimmune conditions, where efficient lymphatic drainage can aid in reducing swelling and promoting tissue repair.

- Balance and Muscle Control: Tai chi emphasizes shifting body weight and maintaining balance, which strengthens the stabilizing muscles and improves coordination. This aspect of tai chi is particularly valuable for women with autoimmune conditions that affect mobility, as it helps prevent falls, improve posture, and promote a sense of physical grounding.

- Energy Flow and Mental Focus: Tai chi is rooted in the concept of Qi (vital energy) and aims to promote its harmonious flow throughout the body. Practitioners focus on mindful, controlled movements that align with their breath, fostering a state of deep relaxation and mental focus. This meditative quality of tai chi can help alleviate mental fatigue, reduce anxiety, and enhance the body's natural resilience against stress-related flare-ups of autoimmune symptoms.

3. Qigong: Harnessing Inner Energy for Healing

Qigong, another traditional Chinese practice, involves a combination of movement, breath control, and meditation aimed at cultivating and balancing the body's internal energy, or Qi. Similar to tai chi, qigong exercises are performed in a slow and controlled manner, emphasizing the connection between mind and body. The practice can be adapted to individual needs, making it an excellent option for women at different stages of their autoimmune health journey.

Research indicates that qigong has the potential to modulate immune function, improve sleep quality, and enhance overall well-being. Studies have shown that regular qigong practice can decrease stress hormones and elevate levels of natural killer (NK) cells, which play a vital role in defending the body against infections and abnormal cellular changes. These immune-regulatory effects are particularly valuable for women with autoimmune conditions, as they support a balanced immune response without provoking inflammation.

- Breathing Techniques: Qigong incorporates deep, diaphragmatic breathing exercises that help expand lung capacity, oxygenate the body, and calm the nervous system. This breathing pattern stimulates the vagus nerve, promoting parasympathetic activity, which in turn reduces the stress-induced release of inflammatory molecules. By fostering a state of relaxation, qigong enables the body to shift its focus from stress response to healing and restoration.

4. Guided Meditation and Mindfulness-Based Stress Reduction (MBSR)

While not involving physical movement, guided meditation and mindfulness-based stress reduction (MBSR) programs complement mind-body exercises like yoga and tai chi. These practices focus on cultivating awareness of the present moment, acknowledging thoughts and emotions without judgment, and fostering a compassionate connection with the body.

MBSR, a structured program that combines mindfulness meditation and gentle movement, has been shown to have profound effects on immune function and inflammation control. Studies indicate that MBSR can lead to a reduction in the production of pro-inflammatory cytokines, particularly in individuals with chronic health conditions. For women with autoimmune diseases, incorporating mindfulness techniques into their daily routine can help manage stress, improve emotional well-being, and support immune regulation.

5. Integrating Mind-Body Practices into Your Routine

The key to reaping the benefits of mind-body exercises lies in consistency and listening to your body's signals. Begin with short, manageable sessions—10-15 minutes per day—and gradually increase the duration as you become more comfortable. The gentle nature of yoga, tai chi, and qigong allows you to adapt the intensity of practice based on how you feel each day, making them suitable components of a long-term wellness plan.

By integrating mind-body exercises into your routine, you can harness their science-backed benefits to promote physical strength, mental clarity, and immune balance. These practices not only alleviate stress but also provide a pathway for women with autoimmune conditions to nurture their bodies, enhance flexibility, and foster a sense of inner peace and resilience.

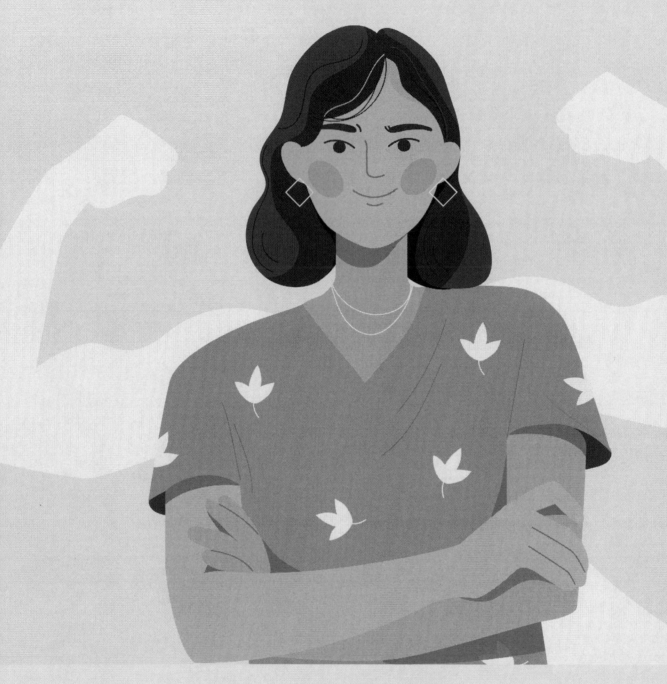

Part III:
Your 60-Day Journey to Feeling Your Best

Chapter 12:
The 60-Day Action Plan

Embarking on a 60-day action plan is a transformative step toward reclaiming your health and well-being. This chapter provides a comprehensive, science-backed blueprint for implementing the Autoimmune Protocol (AIP) diet, tailored to women managing autoimmune conditions. The 60-day plan incorporates the key pillars discussed throughout this book: optimizing nutrition, healing the gut, managing stress, prioritizing sleep, and incorporating mindful physical activity. The timeline is designed to allow gradual dietary and lifestyle changes, offering your body ample time to adapt and respond positively. Each week presents specific goals, strategies, and check-ins to monitor progress, ensuring a personalized approach that aligns with your unique needs. By breaking down the journey into manageable steps, this action plan empowers you to take control of your health, reduce inflammation, and set the foundation for long-term healing. Let's delve into the practical aspects of putting your knowledge into action for a healthier, more vibrant life.

WEEK-BY-WEEK BREAKDOWN OF OBJECTIVES

The following 60-day action plan is divided into week-by-week objectives to help you gradually implement the Autoimmune Protocol (AIP) and lifestyle changes that support optimal immune health. This structure ensures a steady transition, minimizing overwhelm and allowing your body to adapt to dietary and lifestyle shifts. By focusing on specific goals each week, you will build sustainable habits that promote healing, energy, and well-being.

Week 1: Preparation and Mindful Elimination

Objectives:

- Begin by removing gluten, dairy, processed sugars, alcohol, and caffeine from your diet.

- Introduce meal planning and batch cooking using AIP-compliant foods to simplify your routine.

- Start a symptom journal to record daily changes in your physical and emotional state.

Why It Matters: This week sets the stage for your journey by addressing some of the most common inflammatory triggers and preparing your body for deeper dietary adjustments. Logging symptoms helps establish a baseline to measure progress over the following weeks.

Week 2: Deepening the Elimination Phase

Objectives:

- Expand the elimination to include grains, legumes, nuts, seeds, nightshades, and eggs.

- Incorporate a variety of nutrient-dense foods such as leafy greens, root vegetables, wild-caught fish, grass-fed meats, and organ meats.

- Begin incorporating gut-supportive foods like bone broth, fermented vegetables, and coconut kefir to support digestion.

Why It Matters: This week aims to comprehensively remove potential dietary triggers that may contribute to autoimmune flare-ups. By focusing on nutrient-dense foods, you support your body's nutritional needs during this elimination phase, which is critical for tissue repair and immune regulation.

Week 3: Supporting Gut Health and Digestion

Objectives:

- Integrate probiotic and prebiotic foods into your daily meals, such as sauerkraut, kimchi, and fiber-rich vegetables like artichokes and asparagus.

- Practice mindful eating: chew food thoroughly, eat slowly, and avoid distractions during meals.

- Introduce a light evening digestive routine, such as herbal teas (e.g., ginger or peppermint) to promote gut health.

Why It Matters: This week focuses on nurturing your gut microbiome, which plays a central role in immune function and inflammation control. Mindful eating practices enhance digestion and nutrient absorption, aiding in the body's healing processes.

Week 4: Stress Management and Sleep Optimization

Objectives:

- Incorporate daily stress-reduction techniques, such as mindfulness meditation, deep breathing exercises, or journaling for at least 10 minutes each day.

- Establish a consistent sleep schedule, aiming for 7-9 hours of restful sleep per night. Create a bedtime routine that includes screen-free relaxation time.

- Continue tracking symptoms in your journal, noting any correlations between stress levels, sleep quality, and symptom fluctuations.

Why It Matters: Stress and poor sleep are major contributors to immune dysregulation. By prioritizing stress management and sleep, you enhance the body's ability to repair and regulate inflammation, which is crucial for long-term autoimmune management.

Week 5: Incorporating Physical Activity

Objectives:

- Begin integrating gentle, low-impact exercises like walking, yoga, or tai chi into your daily routine, starting with 15-20 minutes and gradually increasing to 30 minutes, 3-4 times a week.

- Monitor your body's response to activity; adjust intensity as needed based on energy levels and symptom feedback.

Why It Matters: Physical activity supports immune function, reduces stress, and promotes joint mobility. Starting with low-impact exercises ensures that your body benefits from movement without provoking inflammation or overexertion.

Week 6: Refining Nutrition and Supporting Micronutrient Intake

Objectives:

- Focus on increasing your intake of micronutrient-rich foods, including sources of zinc, magnesium, vitamin D, and omega-3 fatty acids, such as shellfish, leafy greens, and fatty fish.

- Consider adding supplements if dietary intake is insufficient, after consulting with a healthcare professional.

- Maintain hydration by drinking adequate water throughout the day, aiming for at least 8 cups.

Why It Matters: Optimal intake of key micronutrients is vital for immune health, hormone regulation, and energy production. By prioritizing foods rich in these nutrients, you provide the body with the tools it needs to support healing and vitality.

Week 7: Beginning the Reintroduction Phase

Objectives:

- If you have experienced symptom improvements, begin the reintroduction phase by slowly adding one eliminated food back into your diet every 3-5 days. Start with foods that are least likely to cause reactions, such as certain seeds (e.g., chia seeds) or nuts (e.g., almonds).

- Use your symptom journal to track responses to each reintroduced food, noting any digestive changes, energy shifts, or flare-ups.

- Continue all other lifestyle practices, including stress management, sleep routines, and gentle exercise.

Why It Matters: The reintroduction phase allows you to identify specific food triggers that may contribute to autoimmune symptoms. By approaching this phase systematically, you gain a clearer understanding of your body's tolerances, enabling a more personalized dietary plan moving forward.

Week 8: Reflecting, Adjusting, and Building Long-Term Habits

Objectives:

- Review your symptom journal to identify patterns, triggers, and foods that support or hinder your well-being.

- Create a personalized maintenance plan that includes your reintroduced foods, stress management practices, sleep routines, and physical activities that align with your body's needs.

- Set long-term health goals and strategies for managing potential flare-ups, using the knowledge and habits developed over the past eight weeks.

Why It Matters: Reflecting on your journey helps you understand how dietary and lifestyle changes impact your health. By crafting a personalized maintenance plan, you solidify the habits that support ongoing immune balance, making this 60-day plan the foundation for sustainable wellness.

This week-by-week breakdown provides a structured approach, combining dietary shifts, stress management, sleep optimization, and physical activity. By focusing on small, achievable objectives each week, you progressively build a lifestyle that promotes healing, resilience, and vibrant health.

Chapter 13:
Meal Plans and Delicious Recipes

MEAL PLAN AND RECIPES FOR WEEK 1

	BREAKFAST	LUNCH	SNACK	DINNER	KCAL
DAY 1	SWEET POTATO AND APPLE HASH	AVOCADO CHICKEN SALAD	SLICED CUCUMBERS WITH GUACAMOLE	BAKED SALMON WITH ASPARAGUS	1450 KCAL
DAY 2	BANANA COCONUT SMOOTHIE	TURKEY LETTUCE WRAPS	APPLE SLICES WITH COCONUT BUTTER	ZUCCHINI NOODLES WITH GROUND BEEF	1400 KCAL
DAY 3	COCONUT CHIA PUDDING	AVOCADO TUNA SALAD	CARROT STICKS WITH OLIVE TAPENADE	CHICKEN AND BROCCOLI STIR-FRY	1500 KCAL
DAY 4	BLUEBERRY COCONUT SMOOTHIE	SPINACH AND TURKEY SALAD	BAKED APPLE SLICES WITH CINNAMON	LEMON GARLIC SHRIMP WITH ZUCCHINI NOODLES	1450 KCAL
DAY 5	AVOCADO AND BANANA SMOOTHIE	SARDINE SALAD WITH MIXED GREENS	CARROT AND CUCUMBER STICKS WITH OLIVE TAPENADE	BAKED CHICKEN WITH ROASTED VEGETABLES	1400 KCAL
DAY 6	COCONUT PORRIDGE WITH BERRIES	CHICKEN AND AVOCADO SALAD	BAKED PLANTAIN CHIPS	GARLIC AND HERB BEEF PATTIES WITH STEAMED ASPARAGUS	1500 KCAL
DAY 7	SPINACH AND AVOCADO SMOOTHIE	BAKED COD WITH LEMON AND BROCCOLI	APPLE WITH COCONUT BUTTER	TURKEY ZUCCHINI SKILLET	1450 KCAL

Day 1

Total Calories: ~1450 kcal

Breakfast:

Sweet Potato and Apple Hash

Preparation Time: 5 minutes

Cooking Time: 15 minutes

Servings: 1

Ingredients:

- 1 medium sweet potato, peeled and cubed
- 1 apple, diced
- 1 tbsp coconut oil
- 1/2 tsp cinnamon

Instructions:

1. Heat coconut oil in a skillet over medium heat.

2. Add cubed sweet potato and cook for 10 minutes until softened.

3. Add apple and cinnamon, and cook for another 5 minutes until apples are tender.

Macronutrients: ~250 kcal, 45g carbs, 2g protein, 9g fat

Lunch:

Avocado Chicken Salad

Preparation Time: 10 minutes

Cooking Time: 0 minutes

Servings: 1

Ingredients:

- 1 cooked chicken breast, shredded
- 1/2 avocado, mashed
- 1 tbsp olive oil

- 1/2 lemon, juiced
- 1/2 cup mixed greens

Instructions:

1. In a bowl, mix shredded chicken with mashed avocado, olive oil, and lemon juice.
2. Serve on a bed of mixed greens.

Macronutrients: ~300 kcal, 8g carbs, 30g protein, 18g fat

Snack:

Sliced Cucumbers with Guacamole

Preparation Time: 5 minutes

Cooking Time: 0 minutes

Servings: 1

Ingredients:

- 1/2 cucumber, sliced
- 1/4 avocado, mashed
- 1 tsp olive oil
- Salt to taste

Instructions:

1. Mix mashed avocado, olive oil, and salt to make a quick guacamole.
2. Serve with cucumber slices for dipping.

Macronutrients: ~150 kcal, 10g carbs, 2g protein, 12g fat

Dinner:

Baked Salmon with Asparagus

Preparation Time: 5 minutes

Cooking Time: 20 minutes

Servings: 1

Ingredients:

- 1 salmon fillet
- 5 asparagus spears
- 1 tbsp olive oil
- Salt and herbs to taste

Instructions:

1. Preheat oven to 375°F (190°C).

2. Place salmon and asparagus on a baking sheet. Drizzle with olive oil, salt, and herbs.
3. Bake for 20 minutes until the salmon is cooked through.

Macronutrients: ~750 kcal, 5g carbs, 40g protein, 58g fat

Day 2

Total Calories: ~1400 kcal

Breakfast:

Banana Coconut Smoothie

Preparation Time: 5 minutes

Cooking Time: 0 minutes

Servings: 1

Ingredients:

- 1 banana
- 1/2 cup coconut milk
- 1 tbsp coconut oil

Instructions:

1. Blend all ingredients until smooth.
2. Serve immediately.

Macronutrients: ~300 kcal, 40g carbs, 2g protein, 15g fat

Lunch:

Turkey Lettuce Wraps

Preparation Time: 10 minutes

Cooking Time: 5 minutes

Servings: 1

Ingredients:

- 100g ground turkey
- 1 tbsp olive oil
- 4 large lettuce leaves
- 1/4 cup shredded carrots

Instructions:

1. Cook ground turkey in olive oil over medium heat until fully cooked, about 5 minutes.

2. Spoon turkey onto lettuce leaves and top with shredded carrots.

Macronutrients: ~350 kcal, 10g carbs, 30g protein, 20g fat

Snack:

Apple Slices with Coconut Butter

Preparation Time: 5 minutes

Cooking Time: 0 minutes

Servings: 1

Ingredients:

- 1 apple, sliced
- 1 tbsp coconut butter

Instructions:

1. Slice the apple and spread coconut butter on top.

Macronutrients: ~200 kcal, 30g carbs, 1g protein, 9g fat

Dinner:

Zucchini Noodles with Ground Beef

Preparation Time: 5 minutes

Cooking Time: 10 minutes

Servings: 1

Ingredients:

- 1 zucchini, spiralized
- 100g ground beef
- 1 tbsp olive oil

Instructions:

1. Cook ground beef in olive oil over medium heat for 5 minutes.
2. Add zucchini noodles and cook for an additional 5 minutes until tender.

Macronutrients: ~550 kcal, 10g carbs, 30g protein, 45g fat

Day 3
Total Calories: ~1500 kcal

Breakfast:

Coconut Chia Pudding

Preparation Time: 5 minutes (+overnight soak)

Cooking Time: 0 minutes

Servings: 1

Ingredients:

- 2 tbsp chia seeds
- 1/2 cup coconut milk
- 1 tsp honey

Instructions:

1. Mix chia seeds, coconut milk, and honey in a bowl.
2. Let sit overnight in the fridge.

Macronutrients: ~300 kcal, 20g carbs, 5g protein, 22g fat

Lunch:

Avocado Tuna Salad

Preparation Time: 5 minutes

Cooking Time: 0 minutes

Servings: 1

Ingredients:

- 1 can of tuna, drained
- 1/2 avocado, mashed
- 1 tbsp olive oil

Instructions:

1. Mix tuna, mashed avocado, and olive oil until well combined.

Macronutrients: ~400 kcal, 8g carbs, 28g protein, 30g fat

Snack:

Carrot Sticks with Olive Tapenade

Preparation Time: 5 minutes

Cooking Time: 0 minutes

Servings: 1

Ingredients:

- 1 carrot, cut into sticks
- 2 tbsp olive tapenade

Instructions:

1. Serve carrot sticks with olive tapenade on the side for dipping.

Macronutrients: ~150 kcal, 12g carbs, 1g protein, 11g fat

Dinner:

Chicken and Broccoli Stir-Fry

Preparation Time: 5 minutes

Cooking Time: 15 minutes

Servings: 1

Ingredients:

- 1 chicken breast, diced
- 1 cup broccoli florets
- 1 tbsp coconut oil
- Salt and herbs to taste

Instructions:

1. Heat coconut oil in a pan over medium heat.
2. Add chicken and cook for 10 minutes until browned.
3. Add broccoli and cook for an additional 5 minutes until tender.

Macronutrients: ~650 kcal, 8g carbs, 40g protein, 45g fat

Day 4

Total Calories: ~1450 kcal

Breakfast:

Blueberry Coconut Smoothie

Preparation Time: 5 minutes

Cooking Time: 0 minutes

Servings: 1

Ingredients:

- 1/2 cup blueberries
- 1/2 cup coconut milk
- 1 tbsp coconut oil

Instructions:

1. Blend all ingredients until smooth.
2. Serve immediately.

Macronutrients: ~300 kcal, 20g carbs, 2g protein, 24g fat

Lunch:

Spinach and Turkey Salad

Preparation Time: 10 minutes

Cooking Time: 0 minutes

Servings: 1

Ingredients:

- 100g cooked turkey breast, sliced
- 1 cup spinach leaves
- 1/2 avocado, diced
- 1 tbsp olive oil
- 1/2 lemon, juiced

Instructions:

1. In a bowl, combine spinach, turkey, and avocado.
2. Drizzle with olive oil and lemon juice; mix well.

Macronutrients: ~350 kcal, 10g carbs, 28g protein, 25g fat

Snack:

Baked Apple Slices with Cinnamon

Preparation Time: 5 minutes

Cooking Time: 10 minutes

Servings: 1

Ingredients:

- 1 apple, sliced
- 1/2 tsp cinnamon
- 1 tbsp coconut oil

Instructions:

1. Preheat oven to 350°F (175°C).
2. Coat apple slices with coconut oil and cinnamon.
3. Bake for 10 minutes until tender.

Macronutrients: ~180 kcal, 25g carbs, 1g protein, 10g fat

Dinner:

Lemon Garlic Shrimp with Zucchini Noodles

Preparation Time: 5 minutes

Cooking Time: 10 minutes

Servings: 1

Ingredients:

- 100g shrimp, peeled
- 1 zucchini, spiralized
- 1 tbsp olive oil
- 1/2 lemon, juiced

Instructions:

1. Heat olive oil in a pan over medium heat.
2. Add shrimp and cook for 5 minutes, then add zucchini noodles and lemon juice. Cook for another 5 minutes.

Macronutrients: ~620 kcal, 8g carbs, 35g protein, 48g fat

Day 5
Total Calories: ~1400 kcal

Breakfast:

Avocado and Banana Smoothie

Preparation Time: 5 minutes

Cooking Time: 0 minutes

Servings: 1

Ingredients:

- 1/2 avocado
- 1 banana
- 1/2 cup coconut milk

Instructions:

1. Blend all ingredients until smooth.
2. Serve immediately.

Macronutrients: ~350 kcal, 40g carbs, 3g protein, 22g fat

Lunch:

Sardine Salad with Mixed Greens

Preparation Time: 5 minutes

Cooking Time: 0 minutes

Servings: 1

Ingredients:

- 1 can sardines in olive oil, drained
- 1 cup mixed greens
- 1 tbsp olive oil
- 1/2 lemon, juiced

Instructions:

1. In a bowl, combine sardines and mixed greens.
2. Drizzle with olive oil and lemon juice; mix gently.

Macronutrients: ~350 kcal, 5g carbs, 25g protein, 28g fat

Snack:

Carrot and Cucumber Sticks with Olive Tapenade

Preparation Time: 5 minutes

Cooking Time: 0 minutes

Servings: 1

Ingredients:

- 1 carrot, cut into sticks
- 1/2 cucumber, sliced
- 2 tbsp olive tapenade

Instructions:

1. Serve carrot and cucumber sticks with olive tapenade for dipping.

Macronutrients: ~150 kcal, 10g carbs, 2g protein, 12g fat

Dinner:

Baked Chicken with Roasted Vegetables

Preparation Time: 5 minutes

Cooking Time: 20 minutes

Servings: 1

Ingredients:

- 1 chicken breast
- 1/2 cup broccoli florets
- 1/2 cup carrots, sliced
- 1 tbsp coconut oil

Instructions:

1. Preheat oven to 375°F (190°C).
2. Place chicken, broccoli, and carrots on a baking sheet. Drizzle with melted coconut oil.
3. Bake for 20 minutes until chicken is cooked through.

Macronutrients: ~550 kcal, 15g carbs, 35g protein, 30g fat

Day 6
Total Calories: ~1500 kcal

Breakfast:

Coconut Porridge with Berries

Preparation Time: 5 minutes

Cooking Time: 5 minutes

Servings: 1

Ingredients:

- 1/4 cup coconut flour
- 1/2 cup coconut milk
- 1/4 cup mixed berries
- 1 tbsp honey

Instructions:

1. In a small pot, mix coconut flour and coconut milk. Heat over low, stirring continuously for 5 minutes until thickened.
2. Top with berries and drizzle with honey.

Macronutrients: ~350 kcal, 35g carbs, 4g protein, 20g fat

Lunch:

Chicken and Avocado Salad

Preparation Time: 5 minutes

Cooking Time: 0 minutes

Servings: 1

Ingredients:

- 1 cooked chicken breast, shredded
- 1/2 avocado, diced
- 1 cup mixed greens
- 1 tbsp olive oil

Instructions:

1. Combine chicken, avocado, and mixed greens in a bowl.
2. Drizzle with olive oil and mix well.

Macronutrients: ~400 kcal, 8g carbs, 28g protein, 28g fat

Snack:

Baked Plantain Chips

Preparation Time: 5 minutes

Cooking Time: 15 minutes

Servings: 1

Ingredients:

- 1 green plantain
- 1 tbsp coconut oil
- Salt to taste

Instructions:

1. Preheat oven to 350°F (175°C).
2. Slice plantain thinly, toss with coconut oil, and spread on a baking sheet.
3. Bake for 15 minutes until crispy.

Macronutrients: ~250 kcal, 40g carbs, 1g protein, 10g fat

Dinner:

Garlic and Herb Beef Patties with Steamed Asparagus

Preparation Time: 5 minutes

Cooking Time: 10 minutes

Servings: 1

Ingredients:

- 100g ground beef
- 1 garlic clove, minced
- 5 asparagus spears

- 1 tbsp olive oil

Instructions:

1. Mix ground beef with minced garlic and form into patties.

2. Cook patties in olive oil over medium heat for 5 minutes on each side.

3. Steam asparagus until tender.

Macronutrients: ~500 kcal, 8g carbs, 30g protein, 40g fat

Day 7

Total Calories: ~1450 kcal

<u>Breakfast</u>:

Spinach and Avocado Smoothie

Preparation Time: 5 minutes

Cooking Time: 0 minutes

Servings: 1

Ingredients:

- 1 cup spinach
- 1/2 avocado
- 1/2 cup coconut milk

Instructions:

1. Blend spinach, avocado, and coconut milk until smooth.

2. Serve immediately.

Macronutrients: ~300 kcal, 20g carbs, 4g protein, 24g fat

<u>Lunch</u>:

Baked Cod with Lemon and Broccoli

Preparation Time: 5 minutes

Cooking Time: 15 minutes

Servings: 1

Ingredients:

- 1 cod fillet
- 1 cup broccoli florets
- 1 tbsp olive oil
- 1/2 lemon, sliced

Instructions:

1. Preheat oven to 375°F (190°C).

2. Place cod and broccoli on a baking sheet, drizzle with olive oil, and top with lemon slices.

3. Bake for 15 minutes until cod is flaky.

Macronutrients: ~400 kcal, 8g carbs, 35g protein, 30g fat

<u>Snack</u>:

Apple with Coconut Butter

Preparation Time: 5 minutes

Cooking Time: 0 minutes

Servings: 1

Ingredients:

- 1 apple, sliced
- 1 tbsp coconut butter

Instructions:

1. Slice apple and spread coconut butter on top.

Macronutrients: ~200 kcal, 30g carbs, 1g protein, 9g fat

<u>Dinner</u>:

Turkey Zucchini Skillet

Preparation Time: 5 minutes

Cooking Time: 15 minutes

Servings: 1

Ingredients:

- 100g ground turkey
- 1 zucchini, diced
- 1 tbsp olive oil
- Salt and herbs to taste

Instructions:

1. Heat olive oil in a skillet over medium heat.

2. Add turkey and cook for 10 minutes.

3. Add zucchini and cook for another 5 minutes until tender.

Macronutrients: ~550 kcal, 10g carbs, 30g protein, 40g fat

	BREAKFAST	LUNCH	SNACK	DINNER	KCAL
DAY 1	ROOT VEGETABLE HASH WITH GROUND BEEF	CHICKEN SALAD WITH FERMENTED VEGETABLES	CARROT STICKS WITH BONE BROTH DIP	BAKED COD WITH KALE AND SWEET POTATO	1500 KCAL
DAY 2	COCONUT CHIA PUDDING WITH BERRIES	SALMON AND SPINACH SALAD WITH COCONUT KEFIR DRESSING	APPLE SLICES WITH COCONUT BUTTER	CHICKEN LIVER WITH ROASTED ROOT VEGETABLES	1450 KCAL
DAY 3	BANANA AND SPINACH SMOOTHIE	GROUND BEEF AND KALE BOWL	CUCUMBER SLICES WITH AVOCADO DIP	BAKED CHICKEN THIGHS WITH BUTTERNUT SQUASH	1500 KCAL
DAY 4	SWEET POTATO AND KALE BREAKFAST BOWL	TUNA SALAD WITH FERMENTED VEGETABLES	APPLE WITH COCONUT KEFIR	BAKED TURKEY MEATBALLS WITH ZUCCHINI NOODLES	1450 KCAL
DAY 5	COCONUT YOGURT WITH FRESH BERRIES	SAUTÉED SHRIMP WITH SPINACH AND SWEET POTATO	CUCUMBER AND AVOCADO SLICES	BAKED CHICKEN WITH ROASTED CARROTS AND PARSNIPS	1500 KCAL
DAY 6	APPLE AND SWEET POTATO HASH	GROUND BEEF AND ZUCCHINI STIR-FRY	CARROT STICKS WITH COCONUT KEFIR DIP	SALMON WITH GARLIC SPINACH	1400 KCAL
DAY 7	BANANA AND COCONUT PORRIDGE	TURKEY AND AVOCADO SALAD	APPLE WITH COCONUT BUTTER	BAKED CHICKEN THIGHS WITH CARROT AND PARSNIP MASH	1500 KCAL

Day 1

Total Calories: ~1500 kcal

Breakfast:

Root Vegetable Hash with Ground Beef

Preparation Time: 5 minutes

Cooking Time: 15 minutes

Servings: 1

Ingredients:

- 1/2 sweet potato, cubed
- 1/2 cup butternut squash, cubed
- 100g ground beef
- 1 tbsp coconut oil

Instructions:

Heat coconut oil in a skillet over medium heat.

1. Add ground beef and cook until browned, about 5 minutes.

2. Add sweet potato and squash, cook for 10 minutes until vegetables are tender.

Macronutrients: ~450 kcal, 25g carbs, 30g protein, 28g fat

Lunch:

Chicken Salad with Fermented Vegetables

Preparation Time: 10 minutes

Cooking Time: 0 minutes

Servings: 1

Ingredients:

- 1 cooked chicken breast, shredded

- 1/2 avocado, diced
- 1/2 cup mixed leafy greens
- 2 tbsp fermented vegetables (e.g., sauerkraut)
- 1 tbsp olive oil

Instructions:

1. Combine chicken, avocado, leafy greens, and fermented vegetables in a bowl.
2. Drizzle with olive oil and mix well.

Macronutrients: ~400 kcal, 10g carbs, 28g protein, 30g fat

Snack:

Carrot Sticks with Bone Broth Dip

Preparation Time: 5 minutes

Cooking Time: 5 minutes

Servings: 1

Ingredients:

- 1 carrot, cut into sticks
- 1/2 cup bone broth
- 1 tbsp coconut cream

Instructions:

1. Heat bone broth in a small pot and stir in coconut cream.
2. Use the warm broth mixture as a dip for carrot sticks.

Macronutrients: ~150 kcal, 10g carbs, 5g protein, 10g fat

Dinner:

Baked Cod with Kale and Sweet Potato

Preparation Time: 5 minutes

Cooking Time: 20 minutes

Servings: 1

Ingredients:

- 1 cod fillet
- 1 cup kale leaves
- 1/2 sweet potato, sliced
- 1 tbsp olive oil

Instructions:

1. Preheat oven to 375°F (190°C).
2. Place cod, kale, and sweet potato on a baking sheet. Drizzle with olive oil.
3. Bake for 20 minutes until the cod is flaky and sweet potato is tender.

Macronutrients: ~500 kcal, 30g carbs, 35g protein, 28g fat

Day 2
Total Calories: ~1450 kcal

Breakfast:

Coconut Chia Pudding with Berries

Preparation Time: 5 minutes (+ overnight soak)

Cooking Time: 0 minutes

Servings: 1

Ingredients:

- 2 tbsp chia seeds
- 1/2 cup coconut milk
- 1/4 cup mixed berries
- 1 tsp honey

Instructions:

1. Mix chia seeds, coconut milk, and honey in a bowl.
2. Let sit overnight in the fridge. Top with berries before serving.

Macronutrients: ~300 kcal, 30g carbs, 4g protein, 20g fat

Lunch:

Salmon and Spinach Salad with Coconut Kefir Dressing

Preparation Time: 10 minutes

Cooking Time: 5 minutes

Servings: 1

Ingredients:

- 1 salmon fillet
- 1 cup spinach leaves
- 1 tbsp coconut kefir

- 1/2 avocado, sliced

Instructions:

1. Cook salmon in a pan over medium heat for 5 minutes until flaky.

2. Place spinach and avocado on a plate, top with salmon, and drizzle with coconut kefir.

Macronutrients: ~450 kcal, 12g carbs, 30g protein, 30g fat

Snack:

Apple Slices with Coconut Butter

Preparation Time: 5 minutes

Cooking Time: 0 minutes

Servings: 1

Ingredients:

- 1 apple, sliced
- 1 tbsp coconut butter

Instructions:

1. Slice the apple and spread coconut butter on top.

Macronutrients: ~200 kcal, 30g carbs, 1g protein, 10g fat

Dinner:

Chicken Liver with Roasted Root Vegetables

Preparation Time: 5 minutes

Cooking Time: 15 minutes

Servings: 1

Ingredients:

- 100g chicken liver
- 1/2 cup carrots, chopped
- 1/2 cup parsnips, chopped
- 1 tbsp olive oil

Instructions:

1. Preheat oven to 375°F (190°C).

2. Place chopped vegetables on a baking sheet and drizzle with olive oil. Roast for 15 minutes.

3. In the meantime, cook chicken liver in a pan for 5 minutes until browned.

Macronutrients: ~500 kcal, 30g carbs, 28g protein, 28g fat

Day 3
Total Calories: ~1500 kcal

Breakfast:

Banana and Spinach Smoothie

Preparation Time: 5 minutes

Cooking Time: 0 minutes

Servings: 1

Ingredients:

- 1 banana
- 1 cup spinach
- 1/2 cup coconut milk

Instructions:

1. Blend banana, spinach, and coconut milk until smooth.

2. Serve immediately.

Macronutrients: ~300 kcal, 45g carbs, 3g protein, 15g fat

Lunch:

Ground Beef and Kale Bowl

Preparation Time: 5 minutes

Cooking Time: 10 minutes

Servings: 1

Ingredients:

- 100g ground beef
- 1 cup kale, chopped
- 1 tbsp olive oil
- 1 garlic clove, minced

Instructions:

1. Heat olive oil in a pan over medium heat.

2. Add garlic and cook for 1 minute, then add ground beef and cook until browned.

3. Add kale and cook for another 3-4 minutes until wilted.

Macronutrients: ~450 kcal, 10g carbs, 30g protein, 35g fat

Cucumber Slices with Avocado Dip

Preparation Time: 5 minutes

Cooking Time: 0 minutes

Servings: 1

Ingredients:

- 1/2 cucumber, sliced
- 1/2 avocado, mashed
- 1 tsp lemon juice

Instructions:

1. Mix mashed avocado and lemon juice to make a dip.
2. Serve with cucumber slices.

Macronutrients: ~150 kcal, 12g carbs, 2g protein, 12g fat

Dinner:

Baked Chicken Thighs with Butternut Squash

Preparation Time: 5 minutes

Cooking Time: 20 minutes

Servings: 1

Ingredients:

- 2 chicken thighs
- 1 cup butternut squash, cubed
- 1 tbsp coconut oil

Instructions:

1. Preheat oven to 375°F (190°C).
2. Place chicken thighs and squash on a baking sheet, drizzle with coconut oil.
3. Bake for 20 minutes until chicken is cooked through and squash is tender.

Macronutrients: ~600 kcal, 25g carbs, 35g protein, 35g fat

Day 4

Total Calories: ~1450 kcal

Breakfast:

Sweet Potato and Kale Breakfast Bowl

Preparation Time: 5 minutes

Cooking Time: 15 minutes

Servings: 1

Ingredients:

- 1/2 sweet potato, cubed
- 1 cup kale, chopped
- 1 tbsp coconut oil

Instructions:

1. Heat coconut oil in a skillet over medium heat.
2. Add sweet potato cubes and cook for 10 minutes until soft.
3. Add kale and cook for another 5 minutes until wilted.

Macronutrients: ~350 kcal, 40g carbs, 4g protein, 20g fat

Lunch:

Tuna Salad with Fermented Vegetables

Preparation Time: 5 minutes

Cooking Time: 0 minutes

Servings: 1

Ingredients:

- 1 can of tuna, drained
- 1/2 avocado, mashed
- 2 tbsp fermented vegetables (e.g., sauerkraut)
- 1 cup mixed greens

Instructions:

1. Mix tuna with mashed avocado and fermented vegetables.
2. Serve over a bed of mixed greens.

Macronutrients: ~400 kcal, 10g carbs, 30g protein, 28g fat

Apple with Coconut Kefir

Preparation Time: 5 minutes

Cooking Time: 0 minutes

Servings: 1

Ingredients:

- 1 apple, sliced
- 2 tbsp coconut kefir

Instructions:

1. Slice the apple and dip in coconut kefir.

Macronutrients: ~150 kcal, 30g carbs, 2g protein, 6g fat

Dinner:

Baked Turkey Meatballs with Zucchini Noodles

Preparation Time: 10 minutes

Cooking Time: 20 minutes

Servings: 1

Ingredients:

- 100g ground turkey
- 1 zucchini, spiralized
- 1 garlic clove, minced
- 1 tbsp olive oil

Instructions:

1. Preheat oven to 375°F (190°C). Mix ground turkey with minced garlic and form into meatballs.
2. Bake meatballs for 20 minutes.
3. While meatballs are baking, sauté zucchini noodles in olive oil for 5 minutes.

Macronutrients: ~550 kcal, 10g carbs, 35g protein, 40g fat

Day 5

Total Calories: ~1500 kcal

Breakfast:

Coconut Yogurt with Fresh Berries

Preparation Time: 5 minutes

Cooking Time: 0 minutes

Servings: 1

Ingredients:

- 1/2 cup coconut yogurt
- 1/4 cup mixed berries
- 1 tsp honey

Instructions:

1. Mix coconut yogurt and honey in a bowl.
2. Top with fresh berries and serve.

Macronutrients: ~300 kcal, 30g carbs, 3g protein, 20g fat

Lunch:

Sautéed Shrimp with Spinach and Sweet Potato

Preparation Time: 5 minutes

Cooking Time: 15 minutes

Servings: 1

Ingredients:

- 100g shrimp, peeled
- 1 cup spinach
- 1/2 sweet potato, cubed
- 1 tbsp olive oil

Instructions:

1. Heat olive oil in a pan over medium heat.
2. Add sweet potato cubes and cook for 10 minutes until soft.
3. Add shrimp and spinach, cooking for another 5 minutes until shrimp is pink and spinach wilted.

Macronutrients: ~450 kcal, 35g carbs, 30g protein, 25g fat

Cucumber and Avocado Slices

Preparation Time: 5 minutes

Cooking Time: 0 minutes

Servings: 1

Ingredients:

- 1/2 cucumber, sliced
- 1/2 avocado, sliced

Instructions:

1. Arrange cucumber and avocado slices on a plate and enjoy as a simple snack.

Macronutrients: ~150 kcal, 10g carbs, 2g protein, 12g fat

Dinner:

Baked Chicken with Roasted Carrots and Parsnips

Preparation Time: 5 minutes

Cooking Time: 25 minutes

Servings: 1

Ingredients:

- 1 chicken breast
- 1/2 cup carrots, sliced
- 1/2 cup parsnips, sliced
- 1 tbsp coconut oil

Instructions:

1. Preheat oven to 375°F (190°C).
2. Place chicken breast, carrots, and parsnips on a baking sheet. Drizzle with coconut oil.
3. Bake for 25 minutes until chicken is cooked through and vegetables are tender.

Macronutrients: ~600 kcal, 30g carbs, 35g protein, 35g fat

Day 6
Total Calories: ~1400 kcal

Breakfast:

Apple and Sweet Potato Hash

Preparation Time: 5 minutes

Cooking Time: 10 minutes

Servings: 1

Ingredients:

- 1/2 sweet potato, cubed
- 1 apple, diced
- 1 tbsp coconut oil

Instructions:

1. Heat coconut oil in a skillet over medium heat.
2. Add sweet potato and cook for 5 minutes.
3. Add apple and cook for another 5 minutes until both are tender.

Macronutrients: ~300 kcal, 45g carbs, 2g protein, 15g fat

Lunch:

Ground Beef and Zucchini Stir-Fry

Preparation Time: 5 minutes

Cooking Time: 10 minutes

Servings: 1

Ingredients:

- 100g ground beef
- 1 zucchini, diced
- 1 tbsp olive oil
- Salt and herbs to taste

Instructions:

1. Heat olive oil in a pan over medium heat.
2. Add ground beef and cook for 5 minutes until browned.
3. Add zucchini and cook for another 5 minutes until tender.

Macronutrients: ~450 kcal, 8g carbs, 30g protein, 35g fat

Carrot Sticks with Coconut Kefir Dip

Preparation Time: 5 minutes

Cooking Time: 0 minutes

Servings: 1

Ingredients:

- 1 carrot, cut into sticks
- 2 tbsp coconut kefir

Instructions:

1. Serve carrot sticks with coconut kefir as a dip.

Macronutrients: ~100 kcal, 10g carbs, 1g protein, 8g fat

Dinner:

Salmon with Garlic Spinach

Preparation Time: 5 minutes

Cooking Time: 15 minutes

Servings: 1

Ingredients:

- 1 salmon fillet
- 1 cup spinach
- 1 garlic clove, minced
- 1 tbsp olive oil

Instructions:

1. Heat olive oil in a pan over medium heat.

2. Add salmon and cook for 10 minutes until flaky.

3. Add garlic and spinach to the pan, cook for another 5 minutes until spinach is wilted.

Macronutrients: ~550 kcal, 8g carbs, 35g protein, 38g fat

Day 7

Total Calories: ~1500 kcal

Breakfast:

Banana and Coconut Porridge

Preparation Time: 5 minutes

Cooking Time: 5 minutes

Servings: 1

Ingredients:

- 1/4 cup coconut flour
- 1 banana, mashed
- 1/2 cup coconut milk

Instructions:

1. In a pot, mix coconut flour, banana, and coconut milk.

2. Heat over low for 5 minutes, stirring until thickened.

Macronutrients: ~350 kcal, 50g carbs, 4g protein, 15g fat

Lunch:

Turkey and Avocado Salad

Preparation Time: 5 minutes

Cooking Time: 0 minutes

Servings: 1

Ingredients:

- 100g cooked turkey breast, sliced
- 1/2 avocado, diced
- 1 cup mixed greens
- 1 tbsp olive oil

Instructions:

1. Combine turkey, avocado, and mixed greens in a bowl.

2. Drizzle with olive oil and mix well.

Macronutrients: ~400 kcal, 8g carbs, 30g protein, 28g fat

Apple with Coconut Butter

Preparation Time: 5 minutes

Cooking Time: 0 minutes

Servings: 1

Ingredients:

- 1 apple, sliced
- 1 tbsp coconut butter

Instructions:

1. Slice the apple and spread coconut butter on top.

Macronutrients: ~200 kcal, 30g carbs, 1g protein, 9g fat

Dinner:

Baked Chicken Thighs with Carrot and Parsnip Mash

Preparation Time: 5 minutes

Cooking Time: 25 minutes

Servings: 1

Ingredients:

- 2 chicken thighs
- 1/2 cup carrots, chopped
- 1/2 cup parsnips, chopped
- 1 tbsp coconut oil

Instructions:

1. Preheat oven to 375°F (190°C).
2. Place chicken thighs on a baking sheet, drizzle with coconut oil, and bake for 25 minutes.
3. While chicken is baking, boil carrots and parsnips until tender. Mash and serve alongside the chicken.

Macronutrients: ~550 kcal, 25g carbs, 35g protein, 38g fat

	BREAKFAST	LUNCH	SNACK	DINNER	KCAL
DAY 1	SPINACH AND SAUERKRAUT SCRAMBLE	ARTICHOKE AND CHICKEN SALAD	APPLE SLICES WITH COCONUT YOGURT	BAKED SALMON WITH ASPARAGUS AND KIMCHI	1500 KCAL
DAY 2	COCONUT MILK CHIA PUDDING WITH BERRIES	TURKEY AND AVOCADO WRAPS WITH FERMENTED VEGETABLES	CARROT STICKS WITH COCONUT KEFIR DIP	GROUND BEEF AND GARLIC ASPARAGUS STIR-FRY	1450 KCAL
DAY 3	BANANA SPINACH SMOOTHIE WITH COCONUT KEFIR	SARDINE SALAD WITH ARTICHOKE HEARTS	APPLE WITH SAUERKRAUT	BAKED CHICKEN THIGHS WITH GARLIC-ROASTED BROCCOLI	1500 KCAL
DAY 4	SWEET POTATO AND KIMCHI HASH	SALMON SALAD WITH FERMENTED VEGETABLES	CUCUMBER AND COCONUT YOGURT DIP	GROUND TURKEY STIR-FRY WITH ASPARAGUS	1500 KCAL
DAY 5	COCONUT MILK SMOOTHIE WITH SPINACH AND AVOCADO	CHICKEN AND ARTICHOKE SALAD WITH OLIVE OIL	CARROT STICKS WITH KIMCHI	BAKED COD WITH GARLIC-ROASTED BRUSSELS SPROUTS	1450 KCAL
DAY 6	APPLE AND COCONUT YOGURT BOWL	TURKEY WRAPS WITH SAUERKRAUT AND AVOCADO	CUCUMBER SLICES WITH COCONUT KEFIR	GARLIC SHRIMP WITH ASPARAGUS AND FERMENTED VEGETABLES	1500 KCAL
DAY 7	BANANA AND SPINACH SMOOTHIE WITH COCONUT KEFIR	GROUND BEEF SALAD WITH ARTICHOKE HEARTS	CARROT STICKS WITH KIMCHI	BAKED CHICKEN THIGHS WITH ROASTED BROCCOLI AND GARLIC	1450 KCAL

Day 1

Total Calories: ~1500 kcal

Breakfast:

Spinach and Sauerkraut Scramble

Preparation Time: 5 minutes

Cooking Time: 5 minutes

Servings: 1

Ingredients:

- 1/2 cup spinach, chopped
- 2 tbsp sauerkraut
- 1 tbsp coconut oil
- 1/2 avocado, sliced

Instructions:

1. Heat coconut oil in a skillet over medium heat.

2. Add spinach and sauté for 2-3 minutes until wilted.

3. Mix in sauerkraut and cook for another minute. Serve with avocado slices.

Macronutrients: ~300 kcal, 12g carbs, 4g protein, 28g fat

Lunch:

Artichoke and Chicken Salad

Preparation Time: 10 minutes

Cooking Time: 0 minutes

Servings: 1

Ingredients:

- 1 cooked chicken breast, shredded
- 1/2 cup artichoke hearts, chopped
- 1 cup mixed greens

- 1 tbsp olive oil
- 1 tbsp apple cider vinegar

Instructions:

1. In a bowl, combine chicken, artichoke hearts, and mixed greens.
2. Drizzle with olive oil and apple cider vinegar; toss to mix.

Macronutrients: ~400 kcal, 10g carbs, 30g protein, 28g fat

Snack:

Apple Slices with Coconut Yogurt

Preparation Time: 5 minutes

Cooking Time: 0 minutes

Servings: 1

Ingredients:

- 1 apple, sliced
- 1/4 cup coconut yogurt

Instructions:

1. Serve apple slices with coconut yogurt for dipping.

Macronutrients: ~200 kcal, 30g carbs, 2g protein, 9g fat

Dinner:

Baked Salmon with Asparagus and Kimchi

Preparation Time: 5 minutes

Cooking Time: 15 minutes

Servings: 1

Ingredients:

- 1 salmon fillet
- 5 asparagus spears
- 1 tbsp olive oil
- 2 tbsp kimchi

Instructions:

1. Preheat oven to 375°F (190°C).
2. Place salmon and asparagus on a baking sheet, drizzle with olive oil.
3. Bake for 15 minutes. Serve with kimchi on the side.

Macronutrients: ~600 kcal, 10g carbs, 35g protein, 45g fat

Day 2
Total Calories: ~1450 kcal

Breakfast:

Coconut Milk Chia Pudding with Berries

Preparation Time: 5 minutes (+ overnight soak)

Cooking Time: 0 minutes

Servings: 1

Ingredients:

- 2 tbsp chia seeds
- 1/2 cup coconut milk
- 1/4 cup mixed berries

Instructions:

1. Mix chia seeds and coconut milk in a bowl.
2. Let sit overnight in the fridge. Top with berries before serving.

Macronutrients: ~300 kcal, 25g carbs, 4g protein, 20g fat

Lunch:

Turkey and Avocado Wraps with Fermented Vegetables

Preparation Time: 10 minutes

Cooking Time: 0 minutes

Servings: 1

Ingredients:

1. 2 large lettuce leaves
2. 100g cooked turkey breast, sliced
3. 1/2 avocado, sliced
4. 2 tbsp fermented vegetables (e.g., sauerkraut)

Instructions:

1. Place turkey and avocado slices on lettuce leaves.
2. Add fermented vegetables, roll up, and serve.

Macronutrients: ~400 kcal, 8g carbs, 30g protein, 28g fat

Carrot Sticks with Coconut Kefir Dip

Preparation Time: 5 minutes

Cooking Time: 0 minutes

Servings: 1

Ingredients:

- 1 carrot, cut into sticks
- 2 tbsp coconut kefir

Instructions:

1. Serve carrot sticks with coconut kefir as a dip.

Macronutrients: ~100 kcal, 10g carbs, 1g protein, 8g fat

Dinner:

Ground Beef and Garlic Asparagus Stir-Fry

Preparation Time: 5 minutes

Cooking Time: 10 minutes

Servings: 1

Ingredients:

- 100g ground beef
- 5 asparagus spears, chopped
- 1 garlic clove, minced
- 1 tbsp olive oil

Instructions:

1. Heat olive oil in a pan over medium heat.
2. Add garlic and cook for 1 minute, then add ground beef and cook until browned.
3. Add asparagus and stir-fry for 5 minutes until tender.

Macronutrients: ~550 kcal, 8g carbs, 30g protein, 38g fat

Day 3

Total Calories: ~1500 kcal

Breakfast:

Banana Spinach Smoothie with Coconut Kefir

Preparation Time: 5 minutes

Cooking Time: 0 minutes

Servings: 1

Ingredients:

- 1 banana
- 1 cup spinach
- 1/4 cup coconut kefir
- 1/2 cup coconut milk

Instructions:

1. Blend all ingredients until smooth.
2. Serve immediately.

Macronutrients: ~350 kcal, 45g carbs, 4g protein, 18g fat

Lunch:

Sardine Salad with Artichoke Hearts

Preparation Time: 5 minutes

Cooking Time: 0 minutes

Servings: 1

Ingredients:

- 1 can sardines in olive oil, drained
- 1/2 cup artichoke hearts, chopped
- 1 cup mixed greens
- 1 tbsp olive oil

Instructions:

1. In a bowl, combine sardines, artichoke hearts, and mixed greens.
2. Drizzle with olive oil and mix well.

Macronutrients: ~400 kcal, 8g carbs, 30g protein, 30g fat

Apple with Sauerkraut

Preparation Time: 5 minutes

Cooking Time: 0 minutes

Servings: 1

Ingredients:

- 1 apple, sliced
- 2 tbsp sauerkraut

Instructions:

1. Serve apple slices with sauerkraut on the side.

Macronutrients: ~150 kcal, 30g carbs, 2g protein, 5g fat

Dinner:

Baked Chicken Thighs with Garlic-Roasted Broccoli

Preparation Time: 5 minutes

Cooking Time: 20 minutes

Servings: 1

Ingredients:

- 2 chicken thighs
- 1 cup broccoli florets
- 1 garlic clove, minced
- 1 tbsp coconut oil

Instructions:

1. Preheat oven to 375°F (190°C).
2. Place chicken thighs and broccoli on a baking sheet. Drizzle with coconut oil and sprinkle with minced garlic.
3. Bake for 20 minutes until chicken is cooked through and broccoli is tender.

Macronutrients: ~600 kcal, 10g carbs, 35g protein, 38g fat

Day 4

Total Calories: ~1500 kcal

Breakfast:

Sweet Potato and Kimchi Hash

Preparation Time: 5 minutes

Cooking Time: 10 minutes

Servings: 1

Ingredients:

- 1/2 sweet potato, cubed
- 2 tbsp kimchi
- 1 tbsp coconut oil

Instructions:

1. Heat coconut oil in a skillet over medium heat.
2. Add sweet potato cubes and cook for 10 minutes until soft.
3. Stir in the kimchi and cook for an additional 2 minutes. Serve hot.

Macronutrients: ~350 kcal, 40g carbs, 3g protein, 20g fat

Lunch:

Salmon Salad with Fermented Vegetables

Preparation Time: 10 minutes

Cooking Time: 5 minutes

Servings: 1

Ingredients:

- 1 salmon fillet
- 1 cup mixed greens
- 2 tbsp fermented vegetables (e.g., sauerkraut)
- 1 tbsp olive oil
- 1/2 lemon, juiced

Instructions:

1. Cook salmon in a pan over medium heat for 5 minutes until flaky.
2. In a bowl, combine mixed greens, fermented vegetables, and cooked salmon.
3. Drizzle with olive oil and lemon juice; mix well.

Macronutrients: ~450 kcal, 12g carbs, 30g protein, 30g fat

Snack:

Cucumber and Coconut Yogurt Dip

Preparation Time: 5 minutes

Cooking Time: 0 minutes

Servings: 1

Ingredients:

- 1/2 cucumber, sliced
- 1/4 cup coconut yogurt

Instructions:

1. Serve cucumber slices with coconut yogurt for dipping.

Macronutrients: ~150 kcal, 10g carbs, 2g protein, 10g fat

Dinner:

Ground Turkey Stir-Fry with Asparagus

Preparation Time: 5 minutes

Cooking Time: 15 minutes

Servings: 1

Ingredients:

- 100g ground turkey
- 5 asparagus spears, chopped
- 1 garlic clove, minced
- 1 tbsp olive oil

Instructions:

1. Heat olive oil in a pan over medium heat.

2. Add garlic and ground turkey, cooking until browned, about 5 minutes.

3. Add asparagus and cook for another 10 minutes until tender.

Macronutrients: ~550 kcal, 10g carbs, 35g protein, 38g fat

Day 5

Total Calories: ~1450 kcal

Breakfast:

Coconut Milk Smoothie with Spinach and Avocado

Preparation Time: 5 minutes

Cooking Time: 0 minutes

Servings: 1

Ingredients:

- 1 cup spinach
- 1/2 avocado
- 1/2 cup coconut milk
- 1 tsp honey

Instructions:

1. Blend all ingredients until smooth.

2. Serve immediately.

Macronutrients: ~350 kcal, 20g carbs, 4g protein, 30g fat

Lunch:

Chicken and Artichoke Salad with Olive Oil

Preparation Time: 10 minutes

Cooking Time: 0 minutes

Servings: 1

Ingredients:

- 1 cooked chicken breast, shredded
- 1/2 cup artichoke hearts, chopped
- 1 cup mixed greens
- 1 tbsp olive oil

Instructions:

1. In a bowl, mix chicken, artichoke hearts, and mixed greens.

2. Drizzle with olive oil and toss to combine.

Macronutrients: ~400 kcal, 10g carbs, 30g protein, 28g fat

Snack:

Carrot Sticks with Kimchi

Preparation Time: 5 minutes

Cooking Time: 0 minutes

Servings: 1

Ingredients:

- 1 carrot, cut into sticks
- 2 tbsp kimchi

Instructions:

1. Serve carrot sticks with kimchi on the side.

Macronutrients: ~100 kcal, 10g carbs, 1g protein, 5g fat

Dinner:

Baked Cod with Garlic-Roasted Brussels Sprouts

Preparation Time: 5 minutes

Cooking Time: 20 minutes

Servings: 1

Ingredients:

- 1 cod fillet
- 1 cup Brussels sprouts, halved
- 1 garlic clove, minced
- 1 tbsp coconut oil

Instructions:

1. Preheat oven to 375°F (190°C).
2. Place cod and Brussels sprouts on a baking sheet. Drizzle with coconut oil and sprinkle with minced garlic.
3. Bake for 20 minutes until cod is flaky and Brussels sprouts are crispy.

Macronutrients: ~600 kcal, 12g carbs, 35g protein, 35g fat

Day 6

Total Calories: ~1500 kcal

Breakfast:

Apple and Coconut Yogurt Bowl

Preparation Time: 5 minutes

Cooking Time: 0 minutes

Servings: 1

Ingredients:

- 1 apple, sliced
- 1/4 cup coconut yogurt
- 1 tsp honey

Instructions:

1. Combine apple slices, coconut yogurt, and honey in a bowl.

Macronutrients: ~300 kcal, 35g carbs, 2g protein, 12g fat

Lunch:

Turkey Wraps with Sauerkraut and Avocado

Preparation Time: 10 minutes

Cooking Time: 0 minutes

Servings: 1

Ingredients:

- 2 large lettuce leaves
- 100g cooked turkey breast, sliced
- 1/2 avocado, sliced
- 2 tbsp sauerkraut

Instructions:

1. Lay turkey slices and avocado on lettuce leaves.
2. Add sauerkraut, roll up, and serve.

Macronutrients: ~400 kcal, 10g carbs, 30g protein, 30g fat

Snack:

Cucumber Slices with Coconut Kefir

Preparation Time: 5 minutes

Cooking Time: 0 minutes

Servings: 1

Ingredients:

- 1/2 cucumber, sliced
- 2 tbsp coconut kefir

Instructions:

1. Serve cucumber slices with coconut kefir on the side.

Macronutrients: ~100 kcal, 10g carbs, 1g protein, 8g fat

Dinner:

Garlic Shrimp with Asparagus and Fermented Vegetables

Preparation Time: 5 minutes

Cooking Time: 10 minutes

Servings: 1

Ingredients:

- 100g shrimp, peeled
- 5 asparagus spears, chopped
- 1 garlic clove, minced
- 1 tbsp olive oil
- 2 tbsp fermented vegetables (e.g., kimchi)

Instructions:

1. Heat olive oil in a pan over medium heat.

2. Add garlic and shrimp, cooking until shrimp turns pink, about 5 minutes.

3. Add asparagus and cook for another 5 minutes. Serve with fermented vegetables on the side.

Macronutrients: ~600 kcal, 10g carbs, 30g protein, 38g fat

Day 7
Total Calories: ~1450 kcal

Breakfast:

Banana and Spinach Smoothie with Coconut Kefir

Preparation Time: 5 minutes

Cooking Time: 0 minutes

Servings: 1

Ingredients:

- 1 banana
- 1 cup spinach
- 1/4 cup coconut kefir
- 1/2 cup coconut milk

Instructions:

1. Blend all ingredients until smooth.

2. Serve immediately.

Macronutrients: ~350 kcal, 45g carbs, 4g protein, 18g fat

Lunch:

Ground Beef Salad with Artichoke Hearts

Preparation Time: 10 minutes

Cooking Time: 5 minutes

Servings: 1

Ingredients:

- 100g ground beef
- 1/2 cup artichoke hearts, chopped
- 1 cup mixed greens
- 1 tbsp olive oil

Instructions:

1. Cook ground beef in a pan over medium heat for 5 minutes until browned.

2. In a bowl, combine beef, artichoke hearts, and mixed greens. Drizzle with olive oil and mix well.

Macronutrients: ~450 kcal, 12g carbs, 30g protein, 30g fat

Carrot Sticks with Kimchi

Preparation Time: 5 minutes

Cooking Time: 0 minutes

Servings: 1

Ingredients:

- 1 carrot, cut into sticks
- 2 tbsp kimchi

Instructions:

1. Serve carrot sticks with kimchi on the side.

Macronutrients: ~100 kcal, 10g carbs, 1g protein, 5g fat

Dinner:

Baked Chicken Thighs with Roasted Broccoli and Garlic

Preparation Time: 5 minutes

Cooking Time: 20 minutes

Servings: 1

Ingredients:

- 2 chicken thighs
- 1 cup broccoli florets
- 1 garlic clove, minced
- 1 tbsp coconut oil

Instructions:

1. Preheat oven to 375°F (190°C).
2. Place chicken thighs and broccoli on a baking sheet. Drizzle with coconut oil and sprinkle with minced garlic.
3. Bake for 20 minutes until chicken is cooked through and broccoli is tender.

Macronutrients: ~550 kcal, 12g carbs, 35g protein, 35g fat

	BREAKFAST	LUNCH	SNACK	DINNER	KCAL
DAY 1	BLUEBERRY COCONUT SMOOTHIE	GRILLED CHICKEN AND SPINACH SALAD	APPLE AND COCONUT BUTTER	BAKED SALMON WITH ROASTED VEGETABLES	1500 KCAL
DAY 2	SWEET POTATO BREAKFAST BOWL	SHRIMP AND AVOCADO SALAD	CARROT STICKS WITH COCONUT YOGURT DIP	TURKEY AND ZUCCHINI SKILLET	1450 KCAL
DAY 3	AVOCADO AND SPINACH SMOOTHIE	CHICKEN SALAD WITH FERMENTED VEGETABLES	APPLE AND COCONUT BUTTER	GARLIC SHRIMP WITH ROASTED BROCCOLI	1500 KCAL
DAY 4	SPINACH AND SWEET POTATO HASH	BAKED SALMON SALAD WITH AVOCADO	CARROT STICKS WITH COCONUT YOGURT DIP	GROUND TURKEY STIR-FRY WITH ZUCCHINI	1450 KCAL
DAY 5	COCONUT MILK CHIA PUDDING WITH BERRIES	GRILLED CHICKEN AND ASPARAGUS SALAD	CUCUMBER SLICES WITH COCONUT YOGURT	BAKED COD WITH ROASTED CARROTS	1500 KCAL
DAY 6	BANANA AND SPINACH SMOOTHIE	TURKEY AND AVOCADO SALAD	APPLE SLICES WITH ALMOND BUTTER (AIP-COMPLIANT SUBSTITUTE)	GARLIC SHRIMP WITH SPINACH AND ASPARAGUS	1450 KCAL
DAY 7	AVOCADO AND SPINACH SMOOTHIE	CHICKEN SALAD WITH SAUERKRAUT	CARROT STICKS WITH COCONUT YOGURT	BAKED CHICKEN THIGHS WITH ROASTED BROCCOLI	1500 KCAL

Day 1

Total Calories: ~1500 kcal

Breakfast:

Blueberry Coconut Smoothie

Preparation Time: 5 minutes

Cooking Time: 0 minutes

Servings: 1

Ingredients:

- 1/2 cup blueberries
- 1/2 banana
- 1/2 cup coconut milk
- 1 tbsp coconut oil

Instructions:

1. Combine all ingredients in a blender.

2. Blend until smooth and serve immediately.

Macronutrients: ~300 kcal, 35g carbs, 3g protein, 20g fat

Lunch:

Grilled Chicken and Spinach Salad

Preparation Time: 10 minutes

Cooking Time: 10 minutes

Servings: 1

Ingredients:

- 1 chicken breast
- 2 cups spinach
- 1/2 avocado, sliced
- 1 tbsp olive oil

Instructions:

1. Grill chicken breast for 10 minutes or until cooked through.
2. Place spinach in a bowl, add grilled chicken and avocado slices.
3. Drizzle with olive oil and serve.

Macronutrients: ~400 kcal, 12g carbs, 35g protein, 28g fat

Snack:

Apple and Coconut Butter

Preparation Time: 5 minutes

Cooking Time: 0 minutes

Servings: 1

Ingredients:

- 1 apple, sliced
- 1 tbsp coconut butter

Instructions:

1. Slice the apple and spread coconut butter on top.

Macronutrients: ~200 kcal, 30g carbs, 1g protein, 9g fat

Dinner:

Baked Salmon with Roasted Vegetables

Preparation Time: 5 minutes

Cooking Time: 20 minutes

Servings: 1

Ingredients:

- 1 salmon fillet
- 1 cup mixed vegetables (e.g., zucchini, bell pepper, carrots)
- 1 tbsp olive oil

Instructions:

1. Preheat oven to 375°F (190°C).
2. Place salmon and vegetables on a baking sheet, drizzle with olive oil.
3. Bake for 20 minutes until salmon is flaky and vegetables are tender.

Macronutrients: ~600 kcal, 20g carbs, 35g protein, 38g fat

Day 2
Total Calories: ~1450 kcal

Breakfast:

Sweet Potato Breakfast Bowl

Preparation Time: 5 minutes

Cooking Time: 10 minutes

Servings: 1

Ingredients:

- 1/2 sweet potato, cubed
- 1 tbsp coconut oil
- 1/2 banana, sliced

Instructions:

1. Heat coconut oil in a skillet over medium heat.
2. Add sweet potato cubes and cook for 10 minutes until soft.
3. Top with banana slices and serve warm.

Macronutrients: ~350 kcal, 40g carbs, 3g protein, 20g fat

Lunch:

Shrimp and Avocado Salad

Preparation Time: 10 minutes

Cooking Time: 5 minutes

Servings: 1

Ingredients:

- 100g shrimp, peeled
- 1/2 avocado, diced
- 1 cup mixed greens
- 1 tbsp olive oil

Instructions:

1. Cook shrimp in a pan over medium heat for 5 minutes until pink.
2. In a bowl, combine shrimp, avocado, and mixed greens.
3. Drizzle with olive oil and serve.

Macronutrients: ~400 kcal, 10g carbs, 30g protein, 28g fat

Carrot Sticks with Coconut Yogurt Dip

Preparation Time: 5 minutes

Cooking Time: 0 minutes

Servings: 1

Ingredients:

- 1 carrot, sliced into sticks
- 1/4 cup coconut yogurt

Instructions:

1. Serve carrot sticks with coconut yogurt for dipping.

Macronutrients: ~150 kcal, 12g carbs, 2g protein, 8g fat

Dinner:

Turkey and Zucchini Skillet

Preparation Time: 5 minutes

Cooking Time: 15 minutes

Servings: 1

Ingredients:

- 100g ground turkey
- 1 zucchini, diced
- 1 tbsp olive oil
- Salt and herbs to taste

Instructions:

1. Heat olive oil in a skillet over medium heat.
2. Add ground turkey and cook for 10 minutes until browned.
3. Add zucchini and cook for another 5 minutes until tender.

Macronutrients: ~550 kcal, 10g carbs, 30g protein, 35g fat

Day 3

Total Calories: ~1500 kcal

Breakfast:

Avocado and Spinach Smoothie

Preparation Time: 5 minutes

Cooking Time: 0 minutes

Servings: 1

Ingredients:

- 1/2 avocado
- 1 cup spinach
- 1/2 cup coconut milk
- 1 tsp honey

Instructions:

1. Blend all ingredients until smooth.
2. Serve immediately.

Macronutrients: ~300 kcal, 20g carbs, 4g protein, 25g fat

Lunch:

Chicken Salad with Fermented Vegetables

Preparation Time: 10 minutes

Cooking Time: 0 minutes

Servings: 1

Ingredients:

- 1 cooked chicken breast, shredded
- 2 tbsp fermented vegetables (e.g., sauerkraut)
- 1 cup mixed greens
- 1 tbsp olive oil

Instructions:

1. Combine chicken, fermented vegetables, and mixed greens in a bowl.
2. Drizzle with olive oil and toss to mix.

Macronutrients: ~400 kcal, 10g carbs, 30g protein, 28g fat

Apple and Coconut Butter

Preparation Time: 5 minutes

Cooking Time: 0 minutes

Servings: 1

Ingredients:

- 1 apple, sliced
- 1 tbsp coconut butter

Instructions:

1. Slice the apple and spread coconut butter on top.

Macronutrients: ~200 kcal, 30g carbs, 1g protein, 9g fat

Dinner:

Garlic Shrimp with Roasted Broccoli

Preparation Time: 5 minutes

Cooking Time: 15 minutes

Servings: 1

Ingredients:

- 100g shrimp, peeled
- 1 cup broccoli florets
- 1 garlic clove, minced
- 1 tbsp olive oil

Instructions:

1. Preheat oven to 375°F (190°C).
2. Place shrimp and broccoli on a baking sheet. Drizzle with olive oil and sprinkle with minced garlic.
3. Bake for 15 minutes until shrimp is cooked through and broccoli is tender.

Macronutrients: ~600 kcal, 12g carbs, 30g protein, 38g fat

Day 4

Total Calories: ~1450 kcal

Breakfast:

Spinach and Sweet Potato Hash

Preparation Time: 5 minutes

Cooking Time: 10 minutes

Servings: 1

Ingredients:

- 1/2 sweet potato, cubed
- 1 cup spinach
- 1 tbsp coconut oil

Instructions:

1. Heat coconut oil in a skillet over medium heat.
2. Add sweet potato and cook for 8 minutes until tender.
3. Add spinach and cook for 2 minutes until wilted.

Macronutrients: ~350 kcal, 40g carbs, 3g protein, 20g fat

Lunch:

Baked Salmon Salad with Avocado

Preparation Time: 10 minutes

Cooking Time: 10 minutes

Servings: 1

Ingredients:

- 1 salmon fillet
- 1/2 avocado, sliced
- 1 cup mixed greens
- 1 tbsp olive oil

Instructions:

1. Bake salmon in the oven at 375°F (190°C) for 10 minutes.
2. Combine baked salmon, avocado, and mixed greens in a bowl.
3. Drizzle with olive oil and serve.

Macronutrients: ~400 kcal, 12g carbs, 30g protein, 28g fat

Snack:

Carrot Sticks with Coconut Yogurt Dip

Preparation Time: 5 minutes

Cooking Time: 0 minutes

Servings: 1

Ingredients:

- 1 carrot, sliced into sticks
- 1/4 cup coconut yogurt

Instructions:

1. Serve carrot sticks with coconut yogurt for dipping.

Macronutrients: ~150 kcal, 12g carbs, 2g protein, 8g fat

Dinner:

Ground Turkey Stir-Fry with Zucchini

Preparation Time: 5 minutes

Cooking Time: 15 minutes

Servings: 1

Ingredients:

- 100g ground turkey
- 1 zucchini, diced
- 1 tbsp olive oil

Instructions:

1. Heat olive oil in a skillet over medium heat.

2. Add ground turkey and cook until browned, about 10 minutes.

3. Add zucchini and stir-fry for another 5 minutes until tender.

Macronutrients: ~550 kcal, 10g carbs, 30g protein, 35g fat

Day 5
Total Calories: ~1500 kcal

Breakfast:

Coconut Milk Chia Pudding with Berries

Preparation Time: 5 minutes (+ overnight soak)

Cooking Time: 0 minutes

Servings: 1

Ingredients:

- 2 tbsp chia seeds
- 1/2 cup coconut milk
- 1/4 cup mixed berries

Instructions:

1. Mix chia seeds and coconut milk in a bowl.

2. Let sit overnight in the fridge. Top with berries before serving.

Macronutrients: ~300 kcal, 25g carbs, 4g protein, 20g fat

Lunch:

Grilled Chicken and Asparagus Salad

Preparation Time: 10 minutes

Cooking Time: 10 minutes

Servings: 1

Ingredients:

- 1 chicken breast
- 5 asparagus spears, chopped
- 1 cup mixed greens
- 1 tbsp olive oil

Instructions:

1. Grill chicken breast for 10 minutes until fully cooked.

2. In a bowl, combine mixed greens and asparagus.

3. Slice the grilled chicken and add to the salad, then drizzle with olive oil.

Macronutrients: ~400 kcal, 12g carbs, 35g protein, 28g fat

Snack:

Cucumber Slices with Coconut Yogurt

Preparation Time: 5 minutes

Cooking Time: 0 minutes

Servings: 1

Ingredients:

- 1/2 cucumber, sliced
- 1/4 cup coconut yogurt

Instructions:

1. Serve cucumber slices with coconut yogurt on the side.

Macronutrients: ~100 kcal, 10g carbs, 2g protein, 8g fat

Dinner:

Baked Cod with Roasted Carrots

Preparation Time: 5 minutes

Cooking Time: 20 minutes

Servings: 1

Ingredients:

- 1 cod fillet
- 1 cup carrots, chopped
- 1 tbsp coconut oil

Instructions:

1. Preheat oven to 375°F (190°C).
2. Place cod and carrots on a baking sheet. Drizzle with coconut oil.
3. Bake for 20 minutes until the cod is flaky and carrots are tender.

Macronutrients: ~600 kcal, 15g carbs, 35g protein, 38g fat

Day 6
Total Calories: ~1450 kcal

Breakfast:

Banana and Spinach Smoothie

Preparation Time: 5 minutes

Cooking Time: 0 minutes

Servings: 1

Ingredients:

- 1 banana
- 1 cup spinach
- 1/2 cup coconut milk
- 1 tbsp coconut oil

Instructions:

1. Blend all ingredients until smooth.
2. Serve immediately.

Macronutrients: ~350 kcal, 40g carbs, 3g protein, 25g fat

Lunch:

Turkey and Avocado Salad

Preparation Time: 10 minutes

Cooking Time: 0 minutes

Servings: 1

Ingredients:

- 100g cooked turkey breast, sliced
- 1/2 avocado, diced
- 1 cup mixed greens
- 1 tbsp olive oil

Instructions:

1. In a bowl, mix turkey, avocado, and mixed greens.
2. Drizzle with olive oil and toss to combine.

Macronutrients: ~400 kcal, 10g carbs, 30g protein, 28g fat

Apple Slices with Almond Butter (AIP-Compliant Substitute)

Preparation Time: 5 minutes

Cooking Time: 0 minutes

Servings: 1

Ingredients:

- 1 apple, sliced
- 1 tbsp coconut butter

Instructions:

1. Serve apple slices with coconut butter for dipping.

Macronutrients: ~200 kcal, 30g carbs, 2g protein, 9g fat

Dinner:

Garlic Shrimp with Spinach and Asparagus

Preparation Time: 5 minutes

Cooking Time: 15 minutes

Servings: 1

Ingredients:

- 100g shrimp, peeled
- 1 cup spinach
- 5 asparagus spears, chopped
- 1 tbsp olive oil

Instructions:

1. Heat olive oil in a skillet over medium heat.
2. Add shrimp and cook for 5 minutes until pink.
3. Add spinach and asparagus, cooking for an additional 10 minutes until tender.

Macronutrients: ~500 kcal, 12g carbs, 30g protein, 35g fat

Day 7

Total Calories: ~1500 kcal

Breakfast:

Avocado and Spinach Smoothie

Preparation Time: 5 minutes

Cooking Time: 0 minutes

Servings: 1

Ingredients:

- 1/2 avocado
- 1 cup spinach
- 1/2 cup coconut milk
- 1 tsp honey

Instructions:

1. Blend all ingredients until smooth.
2. Serve immediately.

Macronutrients: ~300 kcal, 20g carbs, 4g protein, 25g fat

Lunch:

Chicken Salad with Sauerkraut

Preparation Time: 10 minutes

Cooking Time: 0 minutes

Servings: 1

Ingredients:

- 1 cooked chicken breast, shredded
- 2 tbsp sauerkraut
- 1 cup mixed greens
- 1 tbsp olive oil

Instructions:

1. Combine chicken, sauerkraut, and mixed greens in a bowl.
2. Drizzle with olive oil and mix well.

Macronutrients: ~400 kcal, 10g carbs, 30g protein, 28g fat

Carrot Sticks with Coconut Yogurt

Preparation Time: 5 minutes

Cooking Time: 0 minutes

Servings: 1

Ingredients:

- 1 carrot, sliced into sticks
- 1/4 cup coconut yogurt

Instructions:

1. Serve carrot sticks with coconut yogurt for dipping.

Macronutrients: ~150 kcal, 12g carbs, 2g protein, 8g fat

Dinner:

Baked Chicken Thighs with Roasted Broccoli

Preparation Time: 5 minutes

Cooking Time: 20 minutes

Servings: 1

Ingredients:

- 2 chicken thighs
- 1 cup broccoli florets
- 1 tbsp coconut oil

Instructions:

1. Preheat oven to 375°F (190°C).

2. Place chicken thighs and broccoli on a baking sheet. Drizzle with coconut oil.

3. Bake for 20 minutes until chicken is cooked through and broccoli is tender.

Macronutrients: ~650 kcal, 15g carbs, 35g protein, 38g fat

	BREAKFAST	LUNCH	SNACK	DINNER	KCAL
DAY 1	SARDINE AND AVOCADO TOAST	SHRIMP AND KALE SALAD	PUMPKIN SEEDS AND BLUEBERRIES	BAKED SALMON WITH SPINACH AND MUSHROOMS	1500 KCAL
DAY 2	SPINACH AND MUSHROOM SCRAMBLE	ZUCCHINI NOODLES WITH CLAMS	CARROT STICKS WITH SUNFLOWER SEED BUTTER	BAKED COD WITH SWISS CHARD AND GARLIC	1450 KCAL
DAY 3	KALE AND AVOCADO SMOOTHIE	SPINACH AND SARDINE SALAD	CELERY STICKS WITH PUMPKIN SEED BUTTER	BAKED MACKEREL WITH ROASTED VEGETABLES	1500 KCAL
DAY 4	CHIA SEED PUDDING WITH COCONUT MILK AND BERRIES	GARLIC SHRIMP WITH BOK CHOY	CUCUMBER SLICES WITH SUNFLOWER SEEDS	BAKED HADDOCK WITH ASPARAGUS	1450 KCAL
DAY 5	SMOKED SALMON AND AVOCADO PLATE	SARDINE AND KALE SALAD	APPLE AND BRAZIL NUTS	BAKED MACKEREL WITH BRUSSELS SPROUTS	1500 KCAL
DAY 6	SPINACH AND MUSHROOM OMELET	TURKEY AND ZUCCHINI STIR-FRY	CUCUMBER SLICES WITH TAHINI	BAKED COD WITH SPINACH AND CARROTS	1450 KCAL
DAY 7	AVOCADO AND SARDINE SALAD	SHRIMP AND SPINACH STIR-FRY	CARROT STICKS WITH HUMMUS (AIP-FRIENDLY)	BAKED SALMON WITH ASPARAGUS AND GARLIC	1500 KCAL

Day 1

Total Calories: ~1500 kcal

Breakfast:

Sardine and Avocado Toast

Preparation Time: 5 minutes

Cooking Time: 0 minutes

Servings: 1

Ingredients:

- 1 small sweet potato, sliced
- 1/2 avocado
- 1 can sardines in olive oil, drained

Instructions:

1. Toast the sweet potato slices until soft.
2. Mash the avocado and spread it on the sweet potato.
3. Top with sardines and serve.

Macronutrients: ~350 kcal, 25g carbs, 15g protein, 22g fat

Lunch:

Shrimp and Kale Salad

Preparation Time: 10 minutes

Cooking Time: 5 minutes

Servings: 1

Ingredients:

- 100g shrimp, peeled
- 2 cups kale, chopped
- 1/2 avocado, diced
- 1 tbsp olive oil

Instructions:

1. Cook shrimp in a pan over medium heat for 5 minutes until pink.

2. In a bowl, combine kale, avocado, and shrimp.

3. Drizzle with olive oil and toss to mix.

Macronutrients: ~400 kcal, 12g carbs, 30g protein, 28g fat

Snack:

Pumpkin Seeds and Blueberries

Preparation Time: 2 minutes

Cooking Time: 0 minutes

Servings: 1

Ingredients:

- 2 tbsp pumpkin seeds
- 1/2 cup blueberries

Instructions:

1. Combine pumpkin seeds and blueberries in a bowl and serve.

Macronutrients: ~200 kcal, 20g carbs, 6g protein, 10g fat

Dinner:

Baked Salmon with Spinach and Mushrooms

Preparation Time: 5 minutes

Cooking Time: 20 minutes

Servings: 1

Ingredients:

- 1 salmon fillet
- 1 cup spinach
- 1/2 cup mushrooms, sliced
- 1 tbsp olive oil

Instructions:

1. Preheat oven to 375°F (190°C).

2. Place salmon, spinach, and mushrooms on a baking sheet. Drizzle with olive oil.

3. Bake for 20 minutes until salmon is cooked through.

Macronutrients: ~550 kcal, 10g carbs, 35g protein, 38g fat

Day 2
Total Calories: ~1450 kcal

Breakfast:

Spinach and Mushroom Scramble

Preparation Time: 5 minutes

Cooking Time: 5 minutes

Servings: 1

Ingredients:

- 1 cup spinach
- 1/2 cup mushrooms, sliced
- 1 tbsp coconut oil

Instructions:

1. Heat coconut oil in a skillet over medium heat.

2. Add spinach and mushrooms, sautéing for 5 minutes until wilted and soft.

Macronutrients: ~300 kcal, 10g carbs, 3g protein, 28g fat

Lunch:

Zucchini Noodles with Clams

Preparation Time: 10 minutes

Cooking Time: 10 minutes

Servings: 1

Ingredients:

- 1 zucchini, spiralized
- 100g canned clams
- 1 garlic clove, minced
- 1 tbsp olive oil

Instructions:

1. Heat olive oil in a pan over medium heat.

2. Add garlic and clams, cooking for 5 minutes.

3. Add zucchini noodles and cook for another 5 minutes until soft.

Macronutrients: ~400 kcal, 15g carbs, 30g protein, 28g fat

Carrot Sticks with
Sunflower Seed Butter

Preparation Time: 5 minutes

Cooking Time: 0 minutes

Servings: 1

Ingredients:

- 1 carrot, sliced into sticks
- 1 tbsp sunflower seed butter

Instructions:

1. Serve carrot sticks with sunflower seed butter for dipping.

Macronutrients: ~200 kcal, 15g carbs, 4g protein, 12g fat

Dinner:

Baked Cod with
Swiss Chard and Garlic

Preparation Time: 5 minutes

Cooking Time: 20 minutes

Servings: 1

Ingredients:

- 1 cod fillet
- 1 cup Swiss chard, chopped
- 1 garlic clove, minced
- 1 tbsp coconut oil

Instructions:

1. Preheat oven to 375°F (190°C).
2. Place cod and Swiss chard on a baking sheet. Drizzle with coconut oil and sprinkle with minced garlic.
3. Bake for 20 minutes until the cod is flaky and Swiss chard is tender.

Macronutrients: ~550 kcal, 10g carbs, 35g protein, 36g fat

Day 3
Total Calories: ~1500 kcal

Breakfast:

Kale and Avocado Smoothie

Preparation Time: 5 minutes

Cooking Time: 0 minutes

Servings: 1

Ingredients:

- 1 cup kale
- 1/2 avocado
- 1/2 cup coconut milk
- 1 tsp honey

Instructions:

1. Blend all ingredients until smooth.
2. Serve immediately.

Macronutrients: ~300 kcal, 20g carbs, 4g protein, 25g fat

Lunch:

Spinach and Sardine Salad

Preparation Time: 10 minutes

Cooking Time: 0 minutes

Servings: 1

Ingredients:

- 1 can sardines in olive oil, drained
- 2 cups spinach
- 1/2 avocado, diced
- 1 tbsp olive oil

Instructions:

1. In a bowl, combine spinach, sardines, and avocado.
2. Drizzle with olive oil and toss to mix.

Macronutrients: ~400 kcal, 12g carbs, 30g protein, 28g fat

Celery Sticks with Pumpkin Seed Butter

Preparation Time: 5 minutes

Cooking Time: 0 minutes

Servings: 1

Ingredients:

- 2 celery stalks
- 1 tbsp pumpkin seed butter

Instructions:

1. Serve celery sticks with pumpkin seed butter for dipping.

Macronutrients: ~150 kcal, 10g carbs, 4g protein, 12g fat

Dinner:

Baked Mackerel with Roasted Vegetables

Preparation Time: 5 minutes

Cooking Time: 20 minutes

Servings: 1

Ingredients:

- 1 mackerel fillet
- 1 cup mixed vegetables (e.g., zucchini, bell pepper, carrot)
- 1 tbsp olive oil

Instructions:

1. Preheat oven to 375°F (190°C).
2. Place mackerel and vegetables on a baking sheet. Drizzle with olive oil.
3. Bake for 20 minutes until the mackerel is cooked through.

Macronutrients: ~650 kcal, 20g carbs, 35g protein, 40g fat

Day 4
Total Calories: ~1450 kcal

Breakfast:

Chia Seed Pudding with Coconut Milk and Berries

Preparation Time: 5 minutes (+ overnight soak)

Cooking Time: 0 minutes

Servings: 1

Ingredients:

- 2 tbsp chia seeds
- 1/2 cup coconut milk
- 1/4 cup mixed berries

Instructions:

1. Mix chia seeds and coconut milk in a bowl.
2. Let sit overnight in the fridge. Top with berries before serving.

Macronutrients: ~300 kcal, 25g carbs, 4g protein, 20g fat

Lunch:

Garlic Shrimp with Bok Choy

Preparation Time: 10 minutes

Cooking Time: 10 minutes

Servings: 1

Ingredients:

- 100g shrimp, peeled
- 1 cup bok choy, chopped
- 1 garlic clove, minced
- 1 tbsp olive oil

Instructions:

1. Heat olive oil in a skillet over medium heat.
2. Add garlic and shrimp, cooking for 5 minutes until pink.
3. Add bok choy and cook for another 5 minutes until tender.

Macronutrients: ~400 kcal, 12g carbs, 30g protein, 28g fat

Cucumber Slices with Sunflower Seeds

Preparation Time: 5 minutes

Cooking Time: 0 minutes

Servings: 1

Ingredients:

- 1/2 cucumber, sliced
- 2 tbsp sunflower seeds

Instructions:

1. Serve cucumber slices with sunflower seeds on the side.

Macronutrients: ~150 kcal, 10g carbs, 4g protein, 10g fat

Dinner:

Baked Haddock with Asparagus

Preparation Time: 5 minutes

Cooking Time: 20 minutes

Servings: 1

Ingredients:

- 1 haddock fillet
- 1 cup asparagus, chopped
- 1 tbsp coconut oil

Instructions:

1. Preheat oven to 375°F (190°C).
2. Place haddock and asparagus on a baking sheet. Drizzle with coconut oil.
3. Bake for 20 minutes until the haddock is flaky and asparagus is tender.

Macronutrients: ~600 kcal, 12g carbs, 35g protein, 36g fat

Day 5
Total Calories: ~1500 kcal

Breakfast:

Smoked Salmon and Avocado Plate

Preparation Time: 5 minutes

Cooking Time: 0 minutes

Servings: 1

Ingredients:

- 100g smoked salmon
- 1/2 avocado, sliced
- 1 tbsp olive oil

Instructions:

1. Arrange smoked salmon and avocado slices on a plate.
2. Drizzle with olive oil and serve.

Macronutrients: ~350 kcal, 10g carbs, 20g protein, 30g fat

Lunch:

Sardine and Kale Salad

Preparation Time: 10 minutes

Cooking Time: 0 minutes

Servings: 1

Ingredients:

- 1 can sardines in olive oil, drained
- 2 cups kale, chopped
- 1/2 avocado, diced
- 1 tbsp lemon juice

Instructions:

1. In a bowl, combine kale, avocado, and sardines.
2. Drizzle with lemon juice and mix well.

Macronutrients: ~400 kcal, 15g carbs, 25g protein, 28g fat

Apple and Brazil Nuts

Preparation Time: 5 minutes

Cooking Time: 0 minutes

Servings: 1

Ingredients:

- 1 apple, sliced
- 3 Brazil nuts

Instructions:

1. Serve apple slices with Brazil nuts on the side.

Macronutrients: ~200 kcal, 30g carbs, 3g protein, 10g fat

Dinner:

Baked Mackerel with Brussels Sprouts

Preparation Time: 5 minutes

Cooking Time: 20 minutes

Servings: 1

Ingredients:

- 1 mackerel fillet
- 1 cup Brussels sprouts, halved
- 1 tbsp coconut oil

Instructions:

1. Preheat oven to 375°F (190°C).
2. Place mackerel and Brussels sprouts on a baking sheet. Drizzle with coconut oil.
3. Bake for 20 minutes until the mackerel is cooked through and sprouts are tender.

Macronutrients: ~550 kcal, 15g carbs, 35g protein, 38g fat

Day 6

Total Calories: ~1450 kcal

Breakfast:

Spinach and Mushroom Omelet

Preparation Time: 5 minutes

Cooking Time: 10 minutes

Servings: 1

Ingredients:

- 2 eggs
- 1 cup spinach
- 1/2 cup mushrooms, sliced
- 1 tbsp coconut oil

Instructions:

1. Heat coconut oil in a skillet over medium heat.
2. Add mushrooms and spinach; cook for 5 minutes.
3. Add eggs and cook until set. Fold in half and serve.

Macronutrients: ~350 kcal, 10g carbs, 20g protein, 30g fat

Lunch:

Turkey and Zucchini Stir-Fry

Preparation Time: 5 minutes

Cooking Time: 10 minutes

Servings: 1

Ingredients:

- 100g ground turkey
- 1 zucchini, diced
- 1 tbsp olive oil
- Salt and pepper to taste

Instructions:

1. Heat olive oil in a skillet over medium heat.
2. Add ground turkey and cook for 5 minutes.
3. Add zucchini and cook for an additional 5 minutes until tender.

Macronutrients: ~400 kcal, 10g carbs, 30g protein, 28g fat

Cucumber Slices with Tahini

Preparation Time: 5 minutes

Cooking Time: 0 minutes

Servings: 1

Ingredients:

- 1/2 cucumber, sliced
- 1 tbsp tahini

Instructions:

1. Serve cucumber slices with tahini for dipping.

Macronutrients: ~150 kcal, 10g carbs, 4g protein, 10g fat

Dinner:

Baked Cod with Spinach and Carrots

Preparation Time: 5 minutes

Cooking Time: 20 minutes

Servings: 1

Ingredients:

- 1 cod fillet
- 1 cup spinach
- 1 carrot, sliced
- 1 tbsp olive oil

Instructions:

1. Preheat oven to 375°F (190°C).

2. Place cod, spinach, and carrot slices on a baking sheet. Drizzle with olive oil.

3. Bake for 20 minutes until the cod is flaky and carrots are tender.

Macronutrients: ~550 kcal, 15g carbs, 35g protein, 36g fat

Day 7

Total Calories: ~1500 kcal

Breakfast:

Avocado and Sardine Salad

Preparation Time: 5 minutes

Cooking Time: 0 minutes

Servings: 1

Ingredients:

- 1 can sardines in olive oil, drained
- 1/2 avocado, sliced
- 1 tbsp lemon juice

Instructions:

1. In a bowl, combine sardines and avocado slices.

2. Drizzle with lemon juice and serve.

Macronutrients: ~350 kcal, 10g carbs, 20g protein, 30g fat

Lunch:

Shrimp and Spinach Stir-Fry

Preparation Time: 5 minutes

Cooking Time: 10 minutes

Servings: 1

Ingredients:

- 100g shrimp, peeled
- 2 cups spinach
- 1 garlic clove, minced
- 1 tbsp olive oil

Instructions:

1. Heat olive oil in a skillet over medium heat.

2. Add garlic and shrimp, cooking for 5 minutes.

3. Add spinach and cook for another 5 minutes until wilted.

Macronutrients: ~400 kcal, 10g carbs, 30g protein, 28g fat

Carrot Sticks with Hummus (AIP-friendly)

Preparation Time: 5 minutes

Cooking Time: 0 minutes

Servings: 1

Ingredients:

- 1 carrot, sliced into sticks
- 2 tbsp AIP-friendly hummus

Instructions:

1. Serve carrot sticks with hummus for dipping.

Macronutrients: ~150 kcal, 15g carbs, 4g protein, 8g fat

Dinner:

Baked Salmon with Asparagus and Garlic

Preparation Time: 5 minutes

Cooking Time: 20 minutes

Servings: 1

Ingredients:

- 1 salmon fillet
- 5 asparagus spears, chopped
- 1 garlic clove, minced
- 1 tbsp coconut oil

Instructions:

1. Preheat oven to 375°F (190°C).
2. Place salmon and asparagus on a baking sheet. Drizzle with coconut oil and sprinkle with minced garlic.
3. Bake for 20 minutes until salmon is cooked through.

Macronutrients: ~600 kcal, 15g carbs, 35g protein, 38g fat

	BREAKFAST	LUNCH	SNACK	DINNER	KCAL
DAY 1	CHIA SEED PUDDING WITH BERRIES (REINTRODUCING CHIA SEEDS)	GRILLED CHICKEN AND AVOCADO SALAD	APPLE SLICES WITH SUNFLOWER SEED BUTTER	BAKED SALMON WITH ROASTED CARROTS AND GARLIC	1500 KCAL
DAY 2	SPINACH AND BANANA SMOOTHIE WITH CHIA SEEDS (REINTRODUCING CHIA SEEDS)	SHRIMP AND AVOCADO SALAD	CARROT STICKS WITH COCONUT YOGURT	BAKED COD WITH ASPARAGUS	1480 KCAL
DAY 3	CHIA SEED PORRIDGE WITH COCONUT MILK (REINTRODUCING CHIA SEEDS)	TURKEY AND MIXED GREENS SALAD WITH ALMONDS (REINTRODUCING ALMONDS)	APPLE SLICES WITH ALMOND BUTTER (REINTRODUCING ALMONDS)	BAKED SALMON WITH ROASTED BRUSSELS SPROUTS	1500 KCAL
DAY 4	AVOCADO AND CHIA SEED SMOOTHIE (CONTINUING WITH CHIA SEEDS)	GRILLED CHICKEN SALAD WITH ALMONDS (REINTRODUCING ALMONDS)	SLICED CUCUMBER WITH SUNFLOWER SEED BUTTER	BAKED MACKEREL WITH ROASTED SWEET POTATOES	1500 KCAL
DAY 5	BANANA AND CHIA SEED PUDDING (CONTINUING WITH CHIA SEEDS)	SHRIMP AND SPINACH SALAD WITH ALMONDS (CONTINUING WITH ALMONDS)	APPLE WITH ALMOND BUTTER (CONTINUING WITH ALMONDS)	BAKED COD WITH ASPARAGUS AND MUSHROOMS	1450 KCAL
DAY 6	SPINACH AND ALMOND SMOOTHIE (CONTINUING WITH ALMONDS)	GRILLED CHICKEN SALAD WITH PUMPKIN SEEDS	CARROT STICKS WITH COCONUT YOGURT	BAKED MACKEREL WITH SWISS CHARD	1480 KCAL
DAY 7	CHIA SEED AND ALMOND BUTTER PUDDING (CONTINUING WITH CHIA SEEDS AND ALMONDS)	TURKEY SALAD WITH MIXED GREENS AND SUNFLOWER SEEDS	BLUEBERRIES WITH COCONUT CREAM	BAKED SALMON WITH SPINACH AND GARLIC	1500 KCAL

Day 1

Total Calories: ~1500 kcal

Breakfast:

Chia Seed Pudding with Berries (Reintroducing Chia Seeds)

Preparation Time: 5 minutes (+ overnight soak)

Cooking Time: 0 minutes

Servings: 1

Ingredients:

- 2 tbsp chia seeds
- 1/2 cup coconut milk
- 1/4 cup mixed berries

Instructions:

1. Mix chia seeds and coconut milk in a bowl.
2. Let sit overnight in the fridge. Top with berries before serving.

Macronutrients: ~300 kcal, 25g carbs, 5g protein, 20g fat

Lunch:

Grilled Chicken and Avocado Salad

Preparation Time: 10 minutes

Cooking Time: 10 minutes

Servings: 1

Ingredients:

- 1 chicken breast
- 2 cups mixed greens
- 1/2 avocado, sliced
- 1 tbsp olive oil

Instructions:

1. Grill the chicken breast for 10 minutes until fully cooked.
2. Place mixed greens in a bowl, add grilled chicken and avocado slices, and drizzle with olive oil.

Macronutrients: ~400 kcal, 12g carbs, 35g protein, 28g fat

Snack:

Apple Slices with Sunflower Seed Butter

Preparation Time: 5 minutes

Cooking Time: 0 minutes

Servings: 1

Ingredients:

- 1 apple, sliced
- 1 tbsp sunflower seed butter

Instructions:

1. Serve apple slices with sunflower seed butter on the side.

Macronutrients: ~200 kcal, 30g carbs, 4g protein, 9g fat

Dinner:

Baked Salmon with Roasted Carrots and Garlic

Preparation Time: 5 minutes

Cooking Time: 20 minutes

Servings: 1

Ingredients:

- 1 salmon fillet
- 1 cup carrots, chopped
- 1 garlic clove, minced
- 1 tbsp olive oil

Instructions:

1. Preheat oven to 375°F (190°C).
2. Place salmon and carrots on a baking sheet, drizzle with olive oil, and sprinkle with minced garlic.
3. Bake for 20 minutes until salmon is cooked through.

Macronutrients: ~600 kcal, 15g carbs, 35g protein, 38g fat

Day 2

Total Calories: ~1480 kcal

Breakfast:

Spinach and Banana Smoothie with Chia Seeds (Reintroducing Chia Seeds)

Preparation Time: 5 minutes

Cooking Time: 0 minutes

Servings: 1

Ingredients:

- 1 cup spinach
- 1/2 banana
- 1/2 cup coconut milk
- 1 tbsp chia seeds

Instructions:

1. Blend all ingredients until smooth.
2. Serve immediately.

Macronutrients: ~300 kcal, 30g carbs, 5g protein, 20g fat

Lunch:

Shrimp and Avocado Salad

Preparation Time: 10 minutes

Cooking Time: 5 minutes

Servings: 1

Ingredients:

- 100g shrimp, peeled
- 2 cups mixed greens
- 1/2 avocado, sliced
- 1 tbsp olive oil

Instructions:

1. Cook shrimp in a pan over medium heat for 5 minutes until pink.
2. Place mixed greens in a bowl, add shrimp and avocado, then drizzle with olive oil.

Macronutrients: ~400 kcal, 12g carbs, 30g protein, 28g fat

Snack:

Carrot Sticks with Coconut Yogurt

Preparation Time: 5 minutes

Cooking Time: 0 minutes

Servings: 1

Ingredients:

- 1 carrot, sliced into sticks
- 1/4 cup coconut yogurt

Instructions:

1. Serve carrot sticks with coconut yogurt for dipping.

Macronutrients: ~150 kcal, 15g carbs, 2g protein, 8g fat

Dinner:

Baked Cod with Asparagus

Preparation Time: 5 minutes

Cooking Time: 20 minutes

Servings: 1

Ingredients:

- 1 cod fillet
- 1 cup asparagus, chopped
- 1 tbsp olive oil

Instructions:

1. Preheat oven to 375°F (190°C).
2. Place cod and asparagus on a baking sheet, drizzle with olive oil, and bake for 20 minutes.

Macronutrients: ~630 kcal, 10g carbs, 35g protein, 32g fat

Day 3

Total Calories: ~1500 kcal

Breakfast:

Chia Seed Porridge with Coconut Milk (Reintroducing Chia Seeds)

Preparation Time: 5 minutes

Cooking Time: 0 minutes

Servings: 1

Ingredients:

- 2 tbsp chia seeds
- 1/2 cup coconut milk
- 1 tsp honey

Instructions:

1. Mix chia seeds and coconut milk in a bowl.
2. Let sit for 10 minutes, stir, then add honey before serving.

Macronutrients: ~300 kcal, 20g carbs, 5g protein, 22g fat

Lunch:

Turkey and Mixed Greens Salad with Almonds (Reintroducing Almonds)

Preparation Time: 10 minutes

Cooking Time: 5 minutes

Servings: 1

Ingredients:

- 100g cooked turkey breast, sliced
- 2 cups mixed greens
- 5 almonds, chopped
- 1 tbsp olive oil

Instructions:

1. In a bowl, mix turkey, mixed greens, and almonds.
2. Drizzle with olive oil and toss to combine.

Macronutrients: ~400 kcal, 15g carbs, 30g protein, 28g fat

Snack:

Apple Slices with Almond Butter (Reintroducing Almonds)

Preparation Time: 5 minutes

Cooking Time: 0 minutes

Servings: 1

Ingredients:

- 1 apple, sliced
- 1 tbsp almond butter

Instructions:

1. Serve apple slices with almond butter on the side.

Macronutrients: ~200 kcal, 30g carbs, 4g protein, 10g fat

Dinner:

Baked Salmon with Roasted Brussels Sprouts

Preparation Time: 5 minutes

Cooking Time: 20 minutes

Servings: 1

Ingredients:

- 1 salmon fillet
- 1 cup Brussels sprouts, halved
- 1 tbsp coconut oil

Instructions:

1. Preheat oven to 375°F (190°C).
2. Place salmon and Brussels sprouts on a baking sheet, drizzle with coconut oil.
3. Bake for 20 minutes until salmon is cooked through.

Macronutrients: ~600 kcal, 15g carbs, 35g protein, 38g fat

Day 4

Total Calories: ~1500 kcal

Breakfast:

Avocado and Chia Seed Smoothie (Continuing with Chia Seeds)

Preparation Time: 5 minutes

Cooking Time: 0 minutes

Servings: 1

Ingredients:

- 1/2 avocado
- 1 cup spinach
- 1/2 cup coconut milk
- 1 tbsp chia seeds

Instructions:

1. Blend all ingredients until smooth.

2. Serve immediately.

Macronutrients: ~300 kcal, 20g carbs, 5g protein, 25g fat

Lunch:

Grilled Chicken Salad with Almonds (Reintroducing Almonds)

Preparation Time: 10 minutes

Cooking Time: 10 minutes

Servings: 1

Ingredients:

- 1 chicken breast
- 2 cups mixed greens
- 1/4 cup sliced almonds
- 1 tbsp olive oil

Instructions:

1. Grill chicken breast for 10 minutes until fully cooked.

2. In a bowl, mix mixed greens and almonds, and top with sliced grilled chicken.

3. Drizzle with olive oil and toss to combine.

Macronutrients: ~400 kcal, 15g carbs, 30g protein, 28g fat

Snack:

Sliced Cucumber with Sunflower Seed Butter

Preparation Time: 5 minutes

Cooking Time: 0 minutes

Servings: 1

Ingredients:

- 1/2 cucumber, sliced
- 1 tbsp sunflower seed butter

Instructions:

1. Serve cucumber slices with sunflower seed butter for dipping.

Macronutrients: ~150 kcal, 10g carbs, 4g protein, 10g fat

Dinner:

Baked Mackerel with Roasted Sweet Potatoes

Preparation Time: 5 minutes

Cooking Time: 20 minutes

Servings: 1

Ingredients:

- 1 mackerel fillet
- 1 cup sweet potato, diced
- 1 tbsp coconut oil

Instructions:

1. Preheat oven to 375°F (190°C).

2. Place mackerel and sweet potato on a baking sheet, drizzle with coconut oil.

3. Bake for 20 minutes until mackerel is cooked through.

Macronutrients: ~650 kcal, 30g carbs, 35g protein, 38g fat

Day 5
Total Calories: ~1450 kcal

Breakfast:

Banana and Chia Seed Pudding (Continuing with Chia Seeds)

Preparation Time: 5 minutes (+ overnight soak)

Cooking Time: 0 minutes

Servings: 1

Ingredients:

- 2 tbsp chia seeds
- 1/2 cup coconut milk
- 1/2 banana, mashed

Instructions:

1. Mix chia seeds, coconut milk, and mashed banana in a bowl.

2. Let sit overnight in the fridge before serving.

Macronutrients: ~300 kcal, 30g carbs, 5g protein, 20g fat

Shrimp and Spinach Salad with Almonds (Continuing with Almonds)

Preparation Time: 10 minutes

Cooking Time: 5 minutes

Servings: 1

Ingredients:

- 100g shrimp, peeled
- 2 cups spinach
- 1/4 cup sliced almonds
- 1 tbsp olive oil

Instructions:

1. Cook shrimp in a pan over medium heat for 5 minutes until pink.

2. In a bowl, combine spinach and shrimp, then top with almonds and drizzle with olive oil.

Macronutrients: ~400 kcal, 15g carbs, 30g protein, 28g fat

Snack:

Apple with Almond Butter (Continuing with Almonds)

Preparation Time: 5 minutes

Cooking Time: 0 minutes

Servings: 1

Ingredients:

- 1 apple, sliced
- 1 tbsp almond butter

Instructions:

1. Serve apple slices with almond butter on the side.

Macronutrients: ~200 kcal, 30g carbs, 4g protein, 10g fat

Dinner:

Baked Cod with Asparagus and Mushrooms

Preparation Time: 5 minutes

Cooking Time: 20 minutes

Servings: 1

Ingredients:

- 1 cod fillet
- 1 cup asparagus, chopped
- 1/2 cup mushrooms, sliced
- 1 tbsp coconut oil

Instructions:

1. Preheat oven to 375°F (190°C).

2. Place cod, asparagus, and mushrooms on a baking sheet. Drizzle with coconut oil.

3. Bake for 20 minutes until cod is flaky and vegetables are tender.

Macronutrients: ~550 kcal, 12g carbs, 35g protein, 36g fat

Day 6

Total Calories: ~1480 kcal

Breakfast:

Spinach and Almond Smoothie (Continuing with Almonds)

Preparation Time: 5 minutes

Cooking Time: 0 minutes

Servings: 1

Ingredients:

- 1 cup spinach
- 1/2 cup coconut milk
- 1/4 cup sliced almonds
- 1 tsp honey

Instructions:

1. Blend all ingredients until smooth.

2. Serve immediately.

Macronutrients: ~300 kcal, 20g carbs, 6g protein, 24g fat

Lunch:

Grilled Chicken Salad with Pumpkin Seeds

Preparation Time: 10 minutes

Cooking Time: 10 minutes

Servings: 1

Ingredients:

- 1 chicken breast
- 2 cups mixed greens
- 2 tbsp pumpkin seeds
- 1 tbsp olive oil

Instructions:

1. Grill chicken breast for 10 minutes until fully cooked.
2. In a bowl, combine mixed greens and pumpkin seeds, then top with sliced grilled chicken.
3. Drizzle with olive oil and toss to combine.

Macronutrients: ~400 kcal, 12g carbs, 30g protein, 28g fat

Snack:

Carrot Sticks with Coconut Yogurt

Preparation Time: 5 minutes

Cooking Time: 0 minutes

Servings: 1

Ingredients:

- 1 carrot, sliced into sticks
- 1/4 cup coconut yogurt

Instructions:

1. Serve carrot sticks with coconut yogurt for dipping.

Macronutrients: ~150 kcal, 12g carbs, 2g protein, 8g fat

Dinner:

Baked Mackerel with Swiss Chard

Preparation Time: 5 minutes

Cooking Time: 20 minutes

Servings: 1

Ingredients:

- 1 mackerel fillet
- 1 cup Swiss chard, chopped
- 1 garlic clove, minced
- 1 tbsp olive oil

Instructions:

1. Preheat oven to 375°F (190°C).
2. Place mackerel and Swiss chard on a baking sheet. Drizzle with olive oil and sprinkle with minced garlic.
3. Bake for 20 minutes until mackerel is cooked through.

Macronutrients: ~630 kcal, 15g carbs, 35g protein, 38g fat

Day 7
Total Calories: ~1500 kcal

Breakfast:

Chia Seed and Almond Butter Pudding
(Continuing with Chia Seeds and Almonds)

Preparation Time: 5 minutes (+ overnight soak)

Cooking Time: 0 minutes

Servings: 1

Ingredients:

- 2 tbsp chia seeds
- 1/2 cup coconut milk
- 1 tbsp almond butter

Instructions:

1. Mix chia seeds, coconut milk, and almond butter in a bowl.
2. Let sit overnight in the fridge before serving.

Macronutrients: ~350 kcal, 20g carbs, 7g protein, 25g fat

Lunch:

Turkey Salad with Mixed Greens and Sunflower Seeds

Preparation Time: 10 minutes

Cooking Time: 0 minutes

Servings: 1

Ingredients:

- 100g cooked turkey breast, sliced
- 2 cups mixed greens
- 2 tbsp sunflower seeds
- 1 tbsp olive oil

Instructions:

1. In a bowl, combine turkey, mixed greens, and sunflower seeds.
2. Drizzle with olive oil and toss to mix.

Macronutrients: ~400 kcal, 15g carbs, 30g protein, 28g fat

Snack:

Blueberries with Coconut Cream

Preparation Time: 5 minutes

Cooking Time: 0 minutes

Servings: 1

Ingredients:

- 1/2 cup blueberries
- 2 tbsp coconut cream

Instructions:

1. Serve blueberries topped with coconut cream.

Macronutrients: ~150 kcal, 18g carbs, 2g protein, 10g fat

Dinner:

Baked Salmon with Spinach and Garlic

Preparation Time: 5 minutes

Cooking Time: 20 minutes

Servings: 1

Ingredients:

- 1 salmon fillet
- 1 cup spinach
- 1 garlic clove, minced
- 1 tbsp coconut oil

Instructions:

1. Preheat oven to 375°F (190°C).
2. Place salmon and spinach on a baking sheet. Drizzle with coconut oil and sprinkle with minced garlic.
3. Bake for 20 minutes until salmon is cooked through.

Macronutrients: ~600 kcal, 12g carbs, 35g protein, 38g fat

WEEK 7: REFLECTING, ADJUSTING, AND BUILDING LONG-TERM HABITS

	BREAKFAST	LUNCH	SNACK	DINNER	KCAL
DAY 1	AVOCADO AND SPINACH SMOOTHIE	BAKED COD WITH MIXED GREENS	APPLE SLICES WITH SUNFLOWER SEED BUTTER	CHICKEN AND SWEET POTATO BAKE	1500 KCAL
DAY 2	CHIA SEED PUDDING WITH BERRIES	GRILLED SALMON SALAD	CARROT STICKS WITH GUACAMOLE	SHRIMP AND ASPARAGUS STIR-FRY	1480 KCAL
DAY 3	SPINACH AND AVOCADO SMOOTHIE BOWL	TURKEY LETTUCE WRAPS	CELERY STICKS WITH SUNFLOWER SEED BUTTER	BAKED MACKEREL WITH STEAMED BROCCOLI	1450 KCAL
DAY 4	COCONUT CHIA SEED PUDDING WITH BANANA SLICES	GRILLED CHICKEN AND AVOCADO SALAD	CARROT STICKS WITH GUACAMOLE	BAKED SALMON WITH ASPARAGUS AND LEMON	1500 KCAL
DAY 5	SPINACH AND AVOCADO SMOOTHIE	SHRIMP AND MIXED GREENS SALAD	APPLE SLICES WITH ALMOND BUTTER (IF REINTRODUCED SUCCESSFULLY)	BAKED COD WITH ROASTED CARROTS	1450 KCAL
DAY 6	COCONUT MILK CHIA PORRIDGE WITH BERRIES	TURKEY AND SPINACH SALAD	SLICED CUCUMBER WITH SUNFLOWER SEED BUTTER	BAKED MACKEREL WITH SWEET POTATOES	1500 KCAL
DAY 7	SPINACH AND BANANA SMOOTHIE	GRILLED CHICKEN AND AVOCADO SALAD	APPLE WITH SUNFLOWER SEED BUTTER	BAKED SALMON WITH BRUSSELS SPROUTS	1500 KCAL

Day 1
Total Calories: ~1500 kcal

Breakfast:

Avocado and Spinach Smoothie

Preparation Time: 5 minutes

Cooking Time: 0 minutes

Servings: 1

Ingredients:
- 1/2 avocado
- 1 cup spinach
- 1/2 cup coconut milk
- 1/2 banana

Instructions:
1. Blend all ingredients until smooth.

2. Serve immediately.

Macronutrients: ~300 kcal, 28g carbs, 5g protein, 22g fat

Lunch:

Baked Cod with Mixed Greens

Preparation Time: 5 minutes

Cooking Time: 20 minutes

Servings: 1

Ingredients:
- 1 cod fillet
- 2 cups mixed greens
- 1 tbsp olive oil
- 1 tbsp lemon juice

Instructions:
1. Preheat oven to 375°F (190°C).

2. Place cod on a baking sheet, drizzle with olive oil and lemon juice, then bake for 20 minutes.

3. Serve with mixed greens.

Macronutrients: ~400 kcal, 12g carbs, 35g protein, 28g fat

Snack:

Apple Slices with Sunflower Seed Butter

Preparation Time: 5 minutes

Cooking Time: 0 minutes

Servings: 1

Ingredients:

- 1 apple, sliced
- 1 tbsp sunflower seed butter

Instructions:

1. Serve apple slices with sunflower seed butter on the side.

Macronutrients: ~200 kcal, 30g carbs, 4g protein, 9g fat

Dinner:

Chicken and Sweet Potato Bake

Preparation Time: 5 minutes

Cooking Time: 25 minutes

Servings: 1

Ingredients:

- 1 chicken breast
- 1 cup sweet potato, diced
- 1 tbsp olive oil
- 1 garlic clove, minced

Instructions:

1. Preheat oven to 375°F (190°C).

2. Place chicken and sweet potatoes on a baking sheet, drizzle with olive oil, and sprinkle with garlic.

3. Bake for 25 minutes until chicken is cooked through.

Macronutrients: ~600 kcal, 35g carbs, 35g protein, 30g fat

Day 2
Total Calories: ~1480 kcal

Breakfast:

Chia Seed Pudding with Berries

Preparation Time: 5 minutes (+ overnight soak)

Cooking Time: 0 minutes

Servings: 1

Ingredients:

- 2 tbsp chia seeds
- 1/2 cup coconut milk
- 1/4 cup mixed berries

Instructions:

1. Mix chia seeds and coconut milk in a bowl.

2. Let sit overnight in the fridge. Top with berries before serving.

Macronutrients: ~300 kcal, 28g carbs, 5g protein, 22g fat

Lunch:

Grilled Salmon Salad

Preparation Time: 10 minutes

Cooking Time: 10 minutes

Servings: 1

Ingredients:

- 1 salmon fillet
- 2 cups mixed greens
- 1/2 avocado, sliced
- 1 tbsp olive oil

Instructions:

1. Grill salmon for 10 minutes until cooked through.

2. In a bowl, mix greens and avocado, top with grilled salmon, and drizzle with olive oil.

Macronutrients: ~450 kcal, 12g carbs, 35g protein, 30g fat

Carrot Sticks with Guacamole

Preparation Time: 5 minutes

Cooking Time: 0 minutes

Servings: 1

Ingredients:

- 1 carrot, sliced into sticks
- 1/4 avocado, mashed
- 1 tsp lemon juice

Instructions:

1. Mix mashed avocado with lemon juice to make guacamole.
2. Serve with carrot sticks.

Macronutrients: ~150 kcal, 15g carbs, 2g protein, 10g fat

Dinner:

Shrimp and Asparagus Stir-Fry

Preparation Time: 5 minutes

Cooking Time: 10 minutes

Servings: 1

Ingredients:

- 100g shrimp, peeled
- 1 cup asparagus, chopped
- 1 tbsp olive oil
- 1 garlic clove, minced

Instructions:

1. Heat olive oil in a pan over medium heat.
2. Add garlic and shrimp, stir-frying for 3 minutes.
3. Add asparagus and cook for another 5 minutes until tender.

Macronutrients: ~580 kcal, 15g carbs, 35g protein, 28g fat

Day 3

Total Calories: ~1450 kcal

Breakfast:

Spinach and Avocado Smoothie Bowl

Preparation Time: 5 minutes

Cooking Time: 0 minutes

Servings: 1

Ingredients:

- 1 cup spinach
- 1/2 avocado
- 1/2 banana
- 1/2 cup coconut milk

Instructions:

1. Blend spinach, avocado, banana, and coconut milk until smooth.
2. Pour into a bowl and serve.

Macronutrients: ~300 kcal, 30g carbs, 5g protein, 22g fat

Lunch:

Turkey Lettuce Wraps

Preparation Time: 10 minutes

Cooking Time: 5 minutes

Servings: 1

Ingredients:

- 100g ground turkey
- 4 large lettuce leaves
- 1/4 avocado, diced
- 1 tbsp olive oil

Instructions:

1. Cook turkey in a pan with olive oil until browned.
2. Place turkey and avocado in lettuce leaves and wrap.

Macronutrients: ~400 kcal, 10g carbs, 30g protein, 28g fat

Celery Sticks with Sunflower Seed Butter

Preparation Time: 5 minutes

Cooking Time: 0 minutes

Servings: 1

Ingredients:

- 2 celery sticks
- 1 tbsp sunflower seed butter

Instructions:

1. Serve celery sticks with sunflower seed butter for dipping.

Macronutrients: ~150 kcal, 10g carbs, 4g protein, 10g fat

Dinner:

Baked Mackerel with Steamed Broccoli

Preparation Time: 5 minutes

Cooking Time: 20 minutes

Servings: 1

Ingredients:

- 1 mackerel fillet
- 1 cup broccoli florets
- 1 tbsp olive oil
- 1 garlic clove, minced

Instructions:

1. Preheat oven to 375°F (190°C).
2. Place mackerel on a baking sheet, drizzle with olive oil, and sprinkle with minced garlic.
3. Bake for 20 minutes while steaming broccoli separately.

Macronutrients: ~600 kcal, 15g carbs, 35g protein, 35g fat

Day 4

Total Calories: ~1500 kcal

Breakfast:

Coconut Chia Seed Pudding with Banana Slices

Preparation Time: 5 minutes (+ overnight soak)

Cooking Time: 0 minutes

Servings: 1

Ingredients:

- 2 tbsp chia seeds
- 1/2 cup coconut milk
- 1/2 banana, sliced

Instructions:

1. Mix chia seeds and coconut milk in a bowl.
2. Let sit overnight in the fridge. Top with banana slices before serving.

Macronutrients: ~320 kcal, 28g carbs, 5g protein, 23g fat

Lunch:

Grilled Chicken and Avocado Salad

Preparation Time: 10 minutes

Cooking Time: 10 minutes

Servings: 1

Ingredients:

- 1 chicken breast
- 2 cups mixed greens
- 1/2 avocado, sliced
- 1 tbsp olive oil

Instructions:

1. Grill chicken breast for 10 minutes until cooked through.
2. In a bowl, combine mixed greens and avocado, then top with sliced grilled chicken.
3. Drizzle with olive oil.

Macronutrients: ~420 kcal, 12g carbs, 35g protein, 28g fat

Snack:

Carrot Sticks with Guacamole

Preparation Time: 5 minutes

Cooking Time: 0 minutes

Servings: 1

Ingredients:

- 1 carrot, sliced into sticks
- 1/4 avocado, mashed
- 1 tsp lime juice

Instructions:

1. Mix mashed avocado with lime juice to make guacamole.
2. Serve with carrot sticks.

Macronutrients: ~150 kcal, 15g carbs, 2g protein, 10g fat

Dinner:

Baked Salmon with Asparagus and Lemon

Preparation Time: 5 minutes

Cooking Time: 20 minutes

Servings: 1

Ingredients:

- 1 salmon fillet
- 1 cup asparagus, trimmed
- 1 tbsp olive oil
- 1 tbsp lemon juice

Instructions:

1. Preheat oven to 375°F (190°C).
2. Place salmon and asparagus on a baking sheet. Drizzle with olive oil and lemon juice.
3. Bake for 20 minutes until salmon is cooked through.

Macronutrients: ~610 kcal, 10g carbs, 35g protein, 38g fat

Day 5

Total Calories: ~1450 kcal

Breakfast:

Spinach and Avocado Smoothie

Preparation Time: 5 minutes

Cooking Time: 0 minutes

Servings: 1

Ingredients:

- 1 cup spinach
- 1/2 avocado
- 1/2 cup coconut milk
- 1/2 banana

Instructions:

1. Blend all ingredients until smooth.
2. Serve immediately.

Macronutrients: ~300 kcal, 28g carbs, 5g protein, 22g fat

Lunch:

Shrimp and Mixed Greens Salad

Preparation Time: 10 minutes

Cooking Time: 5 minutes

Servings: 1

Ingredients:

- 100g shrimp, peeled
- 2 cups mixed greens
- 1 tbsp olive oil
- 1/2 avocado, sliced

Instructions:

1. Cook shrimp in a pan with olive oil for 5 minutes until pink.
2. Combine shrimp, mixed greens, and avocado in a bowl.

Macronutrients: ~420 kcal, 12g carbs, 30g protein, 28g fat

Apple Slices with Almond Butter
(If reintroduced successfully)

Preparation Time: 5 minutes

Cooking Time: 0 minutes

Servings: 1

Ingredients:

- 1 apple, sliced
- 1 tbsp almond butter

Instructions:

1. Serve apple slices with almond butter on the side.

Macronutrients: ~200 kcal, 30g carbs, 4g protein, 10g fat

Dinner:

Baked Cod with Roasted Carrots

Preparation Time: 5 minutes

Cooking Time: 20 minutes

Servings: 1

Ingredients:

- 1 cod fillet
- 1 cup carrots, chopped
- 1 tbsp olive oil
- 1 garlic clove, minced

Instructions:

1. Preheat oven to 375°F (190°C).

2. Place cod and carrots on a baking sheet. Drizzle with olive oil and sprinkle with minced garlic.

3. Bake for 20 minutes until cod is flaky and carrots are tender.

Macronutrients: ~530 kcal, 15g carbs, 35g protein, 32g fat

Day 6
Total Calories: ~1500 kcal

Breakfast:

Coconut Milk Chia Porridge
with Berries

Preparation Time: 5 minutes (+ overnight soak)

Cooking Time: 0 minutes

Servings: 1

Ingredients:

- 2 tbsp chia seeds
- 1/2 cup coconut milk
- 1/4 cup mixed berries

Instructions:

1. Mix chia seeds and coconut milk in a bowl.

2. Let sit overnight in the fridge. Add berries before serving.

Macronutrients: ~320 kcal, 28g carbs, 5g protein, 23g fat

Lunch:

Turkey and Spinach Salad

Preparation Time: 10 minutes

Cooking Time: 5 minutes

Servings: 1

Ingredients:

- 100g turkey breast, cooked and sliced
- 2 cups spinach
- 1 tbsp olive oil
- 1/4 avocado, diced

Instructions:

1. In a bowl, combine turkey, spinach, and avocado.

2. Drizzle with olive oil and mix well.

Macronutrients: ~420 kcal, 10g carbs, 30g protein, 28g fat

Sliced Cucumber with Sunflower Seed Butter

Preparation Time: 5 minutes

Cooking Time: 0 minutes

Servings: 1

Ingredients:

- 1/2 cucumber, sliced
- 1 tbsp sunflower seed butter

Instructions:

1. Serve cucumber slices with sunflower seed butter on the side.

Macronutrients: ~150 kcal, 10g carbs, 4g protein, 10g fat

Dinner:

Baked Mackerel with Sweet Potatoes

Preparation Time: 5 minutes

Cooking Time: 25 minutes

Servings: 1

Ingredients:

- 1 mackerel fillet
- 1 cup sweet potatoes, diced
- 1 tbsp olive oil

Instructions:

1. Preheat oven to 375°F (190°C).
2. Place mackerel and sweet potatoes on a baking sheet. Drizzle with olive oil.
3. Bake for 25 minutes until mackerel is cooked through and sweet potatoes are tender.

Macronutrients: ~610 kcal, 30g carbs, 35g protein, 32g fat

Day 7

Total Calories: ~1500 kcal

Breakfast:

Spinach and Banana Smoothie

Preparation Time: 5 minutes

Cooking Time: 0 minutes

Servings: 1

Ingredients:

- 1 cup spinach
- 1/2 banana
- 1/2 cup coconut milk
- 1 tbsp chia seeds

Instructions:

1. Blend all ingredients until smooth.
2. Serve immediately.

Macronutrients: ~300 kcal, 30g carbs, 5g protein, 22g fat

Lunch:

Grilled Chicken and Avocado Salad

Preparation Time: 10 minutes

Cooking Time: 10 minutes

Servings: 1

Ingredients:

- 1 chicken breast
- 2 cups mixed greens
- 1/2 avocado, sliced
- 1 tbsp olive oil

Instructions:

1. Grill chicken breast for 10 minutes until cooked through.
2. In a bowl, mix greens and avocado, then top with grilled chicken.
3. Drizzle with olive oil.

Macronutrients: ~420 kcal, 12g carbs, 35g protein, 28g fat

Apple with Sunflower Seed Butter

Preparation Time: 5 minutes

Cooking Time: 0 minutes

Servings: 1

Ingredients:

- 1 apple, sliced
- 1 tbsp sunflower seed butter

Instructions:

1. Serve apple slices with sunflower seed butter on the side.

Macronutrients: ~200 kcal, 30g carbs, 4g protein, 9g fat

Dinner:

Baked Salmon with Brussels Sprouts

Preparation Time: 5 minutes

Cooking Time: 20 minutes

Servings: 1

Ingredients:

- 1 salmon fillet
- 1 cup Brussels sprouts, halved
- 1 tbsp olive oil

Instructions:

1. Preheat oven to 375°F (190°C).

2. Place salmon and Brussels sprouts on a baking sheet. Drizzle with olive oil.

3. Bake for 20 minutes until salmon is cooked through.

Macronutrients: ~580 kcal, 15g carbs, 35g protein, 35g fat

Chapter 14:
Navigating Social Situations and Dining Out

Social gatherings and dining out can often present a significant challenge when following the Autoimmune Protocol (AIP) diet. For women managing autoimmune conditions, these scenarios may lead to feelings of isolation or anxiety around food choices. However, with a bit of preparation and a mindful approach, it's possible to enjoy these occasions without compromising your health. This chapter provides science-backed strategies to help you confidently navigate social events, family gatherings, and restaurants while staying true to your AIP lifestyle. We'll discuss ways to communicate your dietary needs effectively, tips for assessing menu options, and methods to manage potential cross-contamination. The goal is to empower you to maintain your dietary boundaries without sacrificing your social life, ensuring a balanced approach to both your health and social well-being. Let's explore practical, adaptable techniques to make your next social outing enjoyable and AIP-friendly.

TIPS FOR EATING OUT WHILE ON AIP

Eating out while following the Autoimmune Protocol (AIP) diet can be challenging, especially when trying to avoid inflammatory triggers and hidden ingredients. However, with a little planning and some key strategies, dining out can still be an enjoyable experience. Here are science-backed tips to help you navigate restaurant menus while maintaining your AIP lifestyle:

1. Do Your Research in Advance: Before choosing a restaurant, look up their menu online to identify potential AIP-friendly dishes. Many establishments now list ingredients and allergens on their websites. Call ahead to ask about their cooking methods and whether they can accommodate your dietary needs, like avoiding certain oils, grains, and nightshades.

2. Stick to Simple Dishes: When in doubt, opt for straightforward meals like grilled meats or seafood paired with steamed vegetables. Avoid dishes with sauces or dressings, as they often contain hidden additives, sugars, or nightshade spices. Request olive oil and lemon wedges on the side to dress your salad or vegetables.

3. Ask for Modifications: Most restaurants are accustomed to making dietary modifications for guests. Politely explain that you have dietary restrictions due to health reasons and ask if certain ingredients can be omitted or substituted. For example, request to have your meal cooked in olive oil instead of vegetable oils or to replace grains with extra vegetables.

4. Bring Your Own Additions: Consider bringing small containers of AIP-friendly foods, such as coconut aminos or your own salad dressing, to enhance your meal without risking exposure to non-compliant ingredients. While this may feel unconventional, many individuals with dietary restrictions find it a practical solution for dining out safely.

5. Communicate Clearly: When ordering, use specific language to communicate your needs. Rather than saying "I can't have dairy," explain that you need your meal to be prepared without butter, cheese, or cream. This level of detail helps the staff understand exactly what to avoid in your dish and reduces the risk of cross-contamination.

6. Select the Right Restaurants: Opt for establishments that focus on fresh, whole foods, such as farm-to-table restaurants or those with a "build-your-own" menu concept. Sushi restaurants can be a good option, where you can order simple sashimi with a side of avocado and steamed vegetables. However, be cautious of soy sauce and other sauces that may contain non-AIP ingredients.

7. Stay Hydrated and Snack Smartly: Drink plenty of water before and during your meal to support digestion and curb potential cravings. If you're unsure about finding AIP-friendly options, consider having a small, AIP-compliant snack before heading out. This approach helps prevent hunger-driven decisions that could lead to dietary compromises.

8. Embrace Flexibility: While it's important to adhere to the AIP diet to manage your autoimmune symptoms, occasional flexibility in social situations is sometimes necessary. If dining out leads to an accidental slip, don't be too hard on yourself. Instead, focus on getting back to your routine immediately after, understanding that a single deviation won't derail your long-term progress.

By employing these strategies, you can confidently navigate eating out while following the AIP diet, making it easier to stay committed to your health goals without missing out on social experiences.

Conclusion

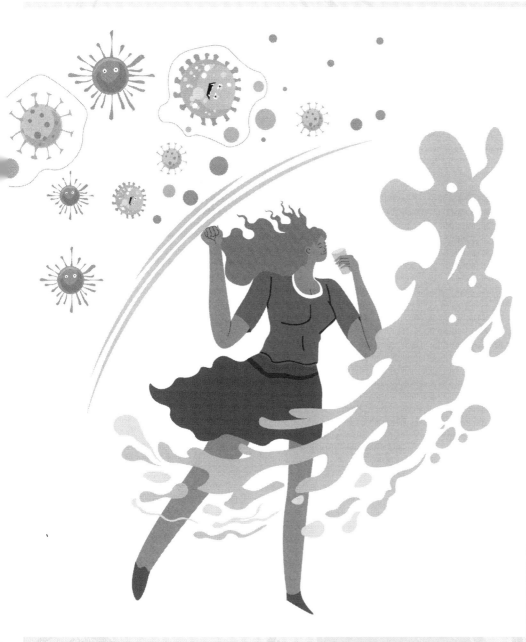

Embarking on the Autoimmune Protocol (AIP) diet is more than a change in eating habits—it is a commitment to your health and well-being. This journey is about reclaiming control over your body and empowering yourself with knowledge to combat the challenges posed by autoimmune conditions. For many women, living with these conditions can feel isolating and unpredictable. Yet, science tells us that with the right approach, it is possible to restore balance and foster healing.

Throughout this book, we've explored the complexities of the immune system, the importance of gut health, and the role diet plays in influencing inflammation and autoimmunity. By adopting the AIP diet, you focus on nutrient-dense foods that support the body's natural healing processes while avoiding potential inflammatory triggers. We've discussed each step of this dietary protocol, from the elimination phase to mindful reintroduction, to help you understand and respond to your body's unique signals.

However, the AIP diet is not just a short-term solution; it's a framework for building sustainable, lifelong habits. By emphasizing whole foods, stress management, adequate sleep, and regular physical activity, you create an environment where your body can thrive. While challenges like dining out and social situations may initially seem daunting, with the strategies provided, you are equipped to navigate these obstacles confidently.

Remember, the goal of the AIP diet is to help you feel your best, to reduce symptoms, and to enhance your quality of life. It's about creating a personalized approach that aligns with your body's needs. Each step you take, each choice you make, brings you closer to understanding how to nourish and support your health from the inside out.

Moving forward, continue to listen to your body and be patient with the process. Healing is not linear, and there will be times when adjustments are necessary. By staying informed, flexible, and mindful, you set the foundation for a healthier future. You have the power to transform your health through the decisions you make every day. This journey is uniquely yours, and it is one you can navigate with strength, knowledge, and resilience.

References

A comprehensive understanding of autoimmune diseases and the Autoimmune Protocol (AIP) diet requires an examination of current scientific research. The information presented in this book has been meticulously curated from peer-reviewed journals, clinical studies, and authoritative sources in the fields of nutrition, immunology, and gut health. The following references provide the scientific foundation for the strategies and dietary guidelines discussed, offering further reading for women interested in delving deeper into the science of autoimmunity and the AIP diet.

1. Ballantyne, S. (2014). The Paleo Approach: Reverse Autoimmune Disease and Heal Your Body. Victory Belt Publishing.

This book serves as a cornerstone in the understanding of the AIP diet, offering a detailed exploration of the mechanisms behind autoimmune conditions and how dietary modifications can impact immune health.

2. Trescott, M., & Alt, A. (2016). The Autoimmune Wellness Handbook: A DIY Guide to Living Well with Chronic Illness. Rodale Books.

A practical guide that synthesizes scientific insights into autoimmune conditions, providing a holistic approach to diet, lifestyle, and emotional well-being.

3. Fasano, A. (2012). Zonulin, regulation of tight junctions, and autoimmune diseases. Annals of the New York Academy of Sciences, 1258(1), 25-33.

This paper introduces the concept of "leaky gut" and its potential role in the development of autoimmune diseases, supporting the AIP diet's emphasis on gut health.

4. Konijeti, G. G., et al. (2017). Efficacy of the Autoimmune Protocol Diet for Inflammatory Bowel Disease. Inflammatory Bowel Diseases, 23(11), 2054-2060.

A clinical study investigating the effects of the AIP diet on patients with inflammatory bowel disease, revealing potential benefits in managing symptoms through dietary changes.

5. Abbott, R. D., Sadowski, A., & Alt, A. G. (2019). Efficacy of the Autoimmune Protocol Diet as Part of a Multi-Disciplinary, Supported Lifestyle Intervention for Hashimoto's Thyroiditis. Cureus, 11(4), e4556.

Research on the impact of the AIP diet on individuals with Hashimoto's thyroiditis, suggesting that dietary interventions can significantly influence quality of life and symptom reduction.

6. Myers, A. (2016). The Autoimmune Solution: Prevent and Reverse the Full Spectrum of Inflammatory Symptoms and Diseases. HarperOne.

This book delves into the mechanisms of autoimmunity, offering an evidence-based perspective on dietary and lifestyle strategies, including the AIP diet, for managing autoimmune diseases.

7. Bischoff, S. C., et al. (2014). Intestinal permeability – a new target for disease prevention and therapy. BMC Gastroenterology, 14(1), 189.

An analysis of intestinal permeability's role in disease development, reinforcing the importance of dietary interventions focused on gut integrity, as advocated in the AIP diet.

8. Clemente, J. C., et al. (2018). The role of the gut microbiome in systemic inflammatory disease. BMJ, 360, j5145.

This study highlights the relationship between gut microbiota and systemic inflammation, supporting the AIP diet's emphasis on nurturing gut health through targeted nutrition.

9. Harvard T.H. Chan School of Public Health. (2020). Nutrition and Immunity.

This resource discusses the link between diet and immune function, underlining how nutrient-dense foods can play a crucial role in supporting a healthy immune system, a principle central to the AIP diet.

10. National Institutes of Health. (2021). Autoimmune Diseases.

A comprehensive overview of autoimmune diseases, providing foundational knowledge about prevalence, mechanisms, and treatment options, framing the context for diet-based interventions like the AIP diet.

11. Vojdani, A. (2014). A potential link between environmental triggers and autoimmunity. Autoimmune Diseases, 2014, 437231.

This paper explores environmental triggers of autoimmunity, emphasizing the potential benefits of dietary modification to reduce exposure to substances that may exacerbate autoimmune symptoms.

12. Lamprecht, M., et al. (2012). Probiotic supplementation affects markers of intestinal barrier, oxidation, and inflammation in trained men; a randomized, double-blinded, placebo-controlled

trial. Journal of the International Society of Sports Nutrition, 9(1), 45.

Research demonstrating the positive effects of probiotics on intestinal barrier function and inflammation, supporting the inclusion of probiotic-rich foods in the AIP diet.

13. Gastroenterology & Hepatology. (2015). The Gut-Immune Connection and its Role in Autoimmunity. Journal of Clinical Investigation.

This review provides insights into the complex interaction between gut health and immune function, lending scientific credence to the AIP diet's focus on dietary changes for immune regulation.

14. Harvard Health Publishing. (2020). Inflammation: A Unifying Theory of Disease.

An examination of how chronic inflammation underlies many health conditions, reinforcing the significance of adopting anti-inflammatory dietary practices, such as those in the AIP protocol.

15. 1National Institute of Allergy and Infectious Diseases (NIAID). (2020). Dietary Approaches to Modulating Autoimmune Diseases.

NIAID's perspective on the role of diet in managing autoimmune diseases, highlighting the potential of the AIP diet as part of a comprehensive lifestyle strategy.

Acknowledging the Sources of Knowledge

The resources listed here represent a blend of clinical evidence, expert insights, and foundational research on autoimmune health. They serve as both a reference point and a springboard for continued learning. In acknowledging these sources, this book aims to provide women with a scientifically robust framework to guide their journey toward improved health through the AIP diet.

About the Author

Eliza Stone is a dedicated advocate for women's health, specializing in autoimmune conditions and the science of nutrition. With a background in clinical nutrition and functional medicine, she has spent over a decade researching the complex interplay between diet, the immune system, and chronic disease. Her focus on the Autoimmune Protocol (AIP) diet stems from a desire to empower women with practical, evidence-based tools to manage their autoimmune symptoms and reclaim their well-being.

After witnessing firsthand the profound impact that dietary changes can have on autoimmune conditions, Eliza Stone made it her mission to translate the latest scientific research into actionable strategies. She combines her expertise in nutritional science with a deep understanding of the unique challenges women face when dealing with autoimmune disorders. Through her work, she aims to demystify the AIP diet, making it accessible and achievable for those seeking relief from inflammation and other autoimmune-related symptoms.

As a published researcher and speaker, Eliza Stone has contributed to the growing body of knowledge on autoimmune health, with particular emphasis on the gut-immune connection, micronutrient therapy, and the role of lifestyle modifications in disease management. She has collaborated with healthcare professionals, nutritionists, and researchers to develop comprehensive protocols that address the root causes of autoimmunity rather than merely treating symptoms.

In addition to her scientific and clinical pursuits, Eliza Stone is a passionate educator. She has led numerous workshops, support groups, and seminars, all aimed at helping women navigate their health journeys with confidence. She understands the emotional and physical toll of autoimmune diseases and strives to provide compassionate guidance alongside evidence-based recommendations.

Eliza Stone believes in a holistic approach to health, one that considers not only diet but also stress management, sleep quality, and physical activity. Her commitment to a science-backed, individualized approach to autoimmune wellness has made her a respected voice in the field. Through this book, she hopes to inspire women to take proactive steps toward healing, using the AIP diet as a foundational tool to support their bodies and enhance their quality of life.

BONUS

HERE IS YOUR FREE GIFT!
SCAN HERE TO DOWNLOAD IT

Made in United States
Orlando, FL
21 December 2024

56351267R00063